Color Atlas
of Histology

Finn Geneser

Color Atlas
of Histology

Munksgaard

Lea & Febiger PHILADELPHIA

Munksgaard

Color Atlas of Histology
1st edition 2nd printing, 1986

Cover and layout by Lars Thorsen
Typesetting: Stibo Sats, Tranbjerg J.
Reproduction: Odense Reproduktion, Odense
Printed in Denmark 1984 by Aarhuus Stiftsbogtrykkerie

ISBN 87-16-09658-4

Distributed in North and South America by

Lea & Febiger
600 S. Washington Square
Philadelphia, PA 19106-4198
(215) 922–1330
U.S.A.

ISBN 0-8121-1052-8

Preface

The purpose of this atlas is to provide *visual* guidance that will make it easy for the student to identify and differentiate between all normal cells, tissues and organs in the human body during practical work with the microscope.

This objective is achieved through the presentation of 428 *color photomicrographs,* each of which has been selected exclusively for its instructive value. Therefore, nearly all the photomicrographs have been made from tissue sections prepared and stained with the methods used in routine histologic and pathologic examination. In addition, each photomicrograph most often demonstrates only one important feature (such as a particular cell or layer) at the magnification commonly used by the student. This has necessitated a large number of small illustrations and is of far more practical help for the student than large pictures that show several details. The latter have only been used for overall orientation in a whole organ and always with appropriate labeling of the relevant structures.

Only photomicrographs are shown, since drawings of tissue sections, although very useful in textbooks, are clearly inferior to high quality photomicrographs when used for the identification of structures in the microscope. Furthermore, only color pictures are shown, since only these fulfil the needs of the unexperienced student.

The illustrations are arranged in chapters in a sequence corresponding to that used in most textbooks and histology courses, and it is expected that the atlas is used in connection with a textbook of histology. Therefore, no line drawings or electron micrographs have been included, and the legend to each illustration deliberately includes only the information that is necessary for the optimal use of that particular illustration in practical microscopy.

I am indebted to many collegues for their generous help with material for some of the illustrations. My sincere thanks are due to Dr. K.T. Drzewiecki, Department of Plastic Surgery, The Finsen Institute, University of Copenhagen (Fig. 11-7), Dr. J. Hastrup and Dr. N.O. Jacobsen, Institute of Pathology, University of Aarhus (Figs 16-23 and 16-24), Dr. U.V. Henriques, Institute of Pathology, University of Aarhus (Fig. 15-16), Dr. J.P. Kroustrup, Institute of Anatomy C, University of Aarhus (Figs 12-32 and 12-52 to 12-55), Dr. L. Malinovský, Department of Anatomy, Purkinje University, Brno (Figs 8-22 to 8-24), Dr. M.M. Matthiessen, Institute of Anatomy A, University of Copenhagen (Figs 12-16 and 12-17), Dr. E. Mortensen, The Central Laboratory, The Municipal Hospital of Aarhus (Figs 5-2 to 5-8 and 5-12 to 5-20), Dr. M. Møller, Institute of Anatomy B, University of Copenhagen (Figs 15-8, 15-10 and 15-11), Dr. S. Seier Poulsen, Institute of Anatomy B, University of Copenhagen (Figs 3-5, 3-6, 12-23, 12-27, 12-29, 12-33, 12-35 to 12-38, 12-42 and 12-43), Dr. N.E. Skakkebæk, Department of Pediatrics, Hvidovre Hospital, Copenhagen (Figs 16-26, 16-27 and 16-29) and Dr. J. Zimmer, Institute of Anatomy B, University of Aarhus (Figs 8-8 to 8-10).

Finally, I offer my most deeply felt thanks to three people in particular, who have been my closest collaborators throughout the work: laboratory technician **Pylle Clausen,** who prepared nearly all the microscopical sections, medical photographer **Albert Meier,** who carried out all the photographical work, and secretary **Karin Wiedemann,** who did all the typing, helped with proofreading and prepared the index. All three of them – by their outstanding care and technical skill – have contributed decisively to the creation of this atlas!

Aarhus, June 1984

Finn Geneser

In the production of this volume, the illustrations have been further improved upon.

Aarhus, August 1985

Finn Geneser

Contents

CHAPTER 1
The Cell

Parietal cells   Chief cells

Oocyte
Cytoplasm   Nucleus   Granulosa cells

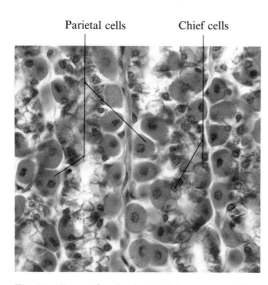

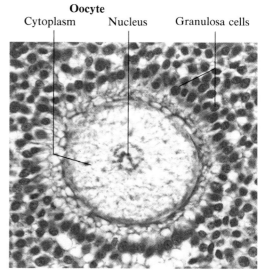

Fig. 1-1. Corpus-fundic glands of the **mucosa of the stomach.** The parietal cells with eosinophilic (red stained) cytoplasm and the chief cells with basophilic (blue stained) cytoplasm are characteristic examples of the general appearance of cells in hematoxylin and eosin (H and E) stained histological sections. H and E. x440.

Fig. 1-2. Oocyte surrounded by granulosa cells in **growing follicle of the ovary,** illustrating the great variation in cell size in the human body. Azan staining. x340.

Branches of dendritic tree

Nuclei   Smooth muscle cells   Cytoplasm

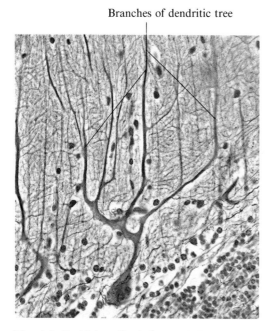

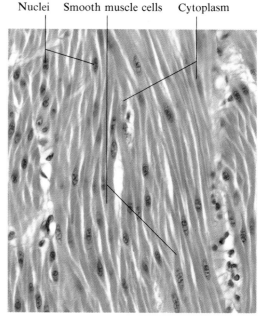

Fig. 1-3. Purkinje cell of the **cerebellar cortex.** Many cells have a very complex shape and the Purkinje cell, with its extensively branched dendritic tree, illustrates this beautifully. Cajal staining. x275.

Fig. 1-4. Smooth muscle cells of the wall of the **small intestine.** Muscle cells are characteristic examples of cells with an elongate shape. H and E. x440.

Cell membrane

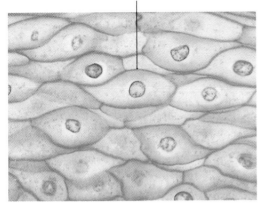

Mitochondria

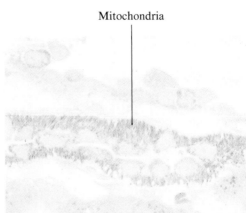

Fig. 1-5. Stratified squamous epithelium of the **esophagus.** The cell membranes are seen distinctly. Van Gieson staining. x660.

Fig. 1-6. Mitochondria in cells of the **proximal tubules of the kidney.** Staining of the mitochondria is due to histochemical demonstration of the enzyme cytochromoxidase which occurs exclusively in mitochondria. x660.

Pancreatic acini Ergastoplasm

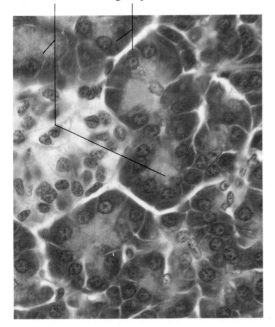

Motor neuron Nissl bodies

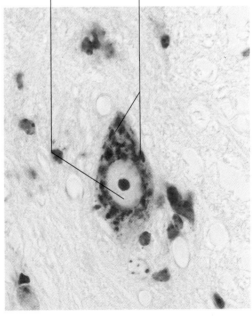

Fig. 1-7. Acini of the **exocrine pancreas.** The acinar gland cells show extensive basophilia in their basal cytoplasm due to the presence of a very well developed ergastoplasm containing ribonucleoprotein. H and E. x660.

Fig. 1-8. Motor neuron in the **anterior horn of the spinal cord.** The ergastoplasm in nerve cells forms characteristic clumps, termed Nissl bodies. Thionine staining. x660.

Negative Golgi image

Golgi apparatus

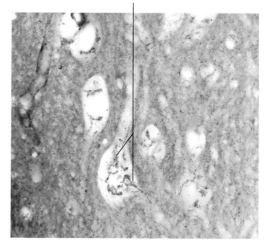

Fig. 1-9. Plasma cells in **lamina propria of the small intestine.** The clear cytoplasmic zone close to the nucleus in some of the plasma cells is a so-called negative Golgi image. It is caused by the contrast between the unstained Golgi apparatus and the surrounding basophilic cytoplasm. H and E. x660.

Fig. 1-10. Golgi apparatus in **neurons of the brain stem.** The section has been fixed in a dichromate solution and then treated with a silver salt (Golgi's original method). The Golgi apparatus in neurons typically surrounds the nucleus and sends extensions into the processes. x660.

Pancreatic acini   Secretory granules   Secretory granules   Pancreatic acini

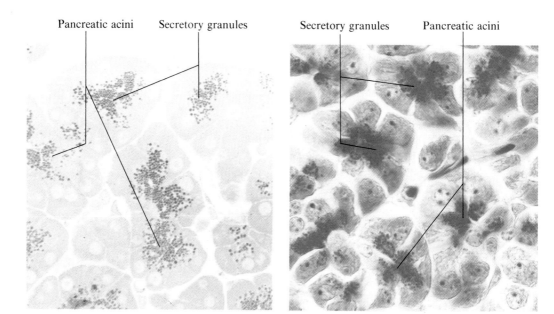

Fig. 1-11. Acini of the **exocrine pancreas.** The apical cytoplasm of the gland cells contains numerous secretory granules. Epon-embedded section stained with methylene blue. x660.

Fig. 1-12. Secretory granules in acinar cells of the **exocrine pancreas.** In this section, the secretory granules are stained bright red. Liisberg's trichrome method. x660.

Lysosomes   Proximal tubules

Sympathetic ganglion cell   Lipofuscin granules

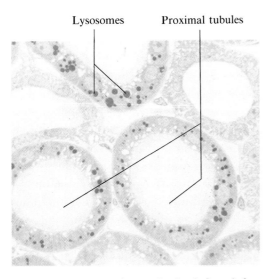

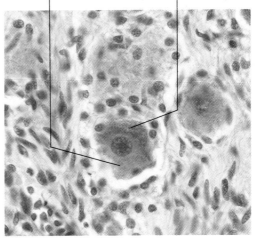

Fig. 1-13. Lysosomes in **proximal tubules of the kidney.** The lysosomes are very large and abundant in these cells. Epon-embedded section stained with methylene blue. x660.

Fig. 1-14. Lipofuscin granules (residual bodies) in **sympathetic ganglion cell.** The golden brown lipofuscin granules are an example of an endogenous pigment inclusion. H and E. x440.

Glycogen granules   Liver cells   Liver cells   Glycogen granules

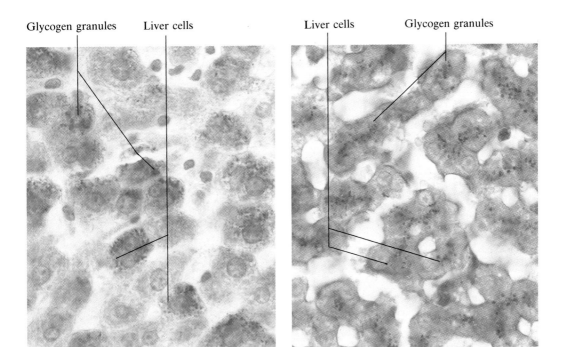

Fig. 1-15. Glycogen granules in **liver cells,** stained bright red with lithium carmine. x660.

Fig. 1-16. Glycogen granules in **liver cells,** stained magenta red using the PAS reaction. x660.

Lipid   Fat cells   Coal dust particles   Macrophages

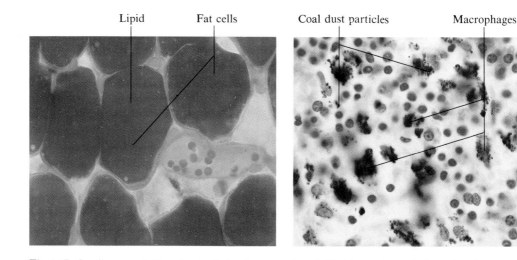

Fig. 1-17. Small accumulation of **fat cells** (unilocular adipose cells). The lipid content of the fat cells has been preserved by cutting frozen sections and is stained red with sudan red (the section is counterstained with Light Green). x440.

Fig. 1-18. Macrophages in **bronchial lymph node.** The macrophages are filled with engulfed coal dust particles. The latter are an example of an exogenous pigment inclusion. H and E. x540.

Melanin granules in cells   Melanocytes loaded   Liver cell nuclei   Endothelial cell nucleus
of posterior epithelium   with melanin granules   Chromatin   Nucleolus   Nucleolemma

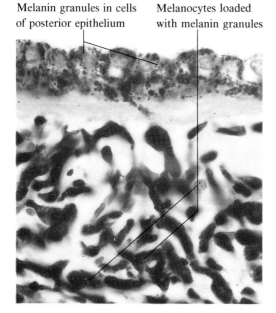   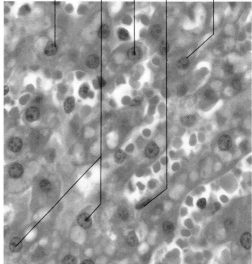

Fig. 1-19. Melanin granules in melanocytes and posterior epithelium of the **iris.** H and E. x660.

Fig. 1-20. Part of **liver lobule** with cords of liver cells. The liver cell nuclei show the characteristic appearance of the nuclear organelles in histological sections. Note also the rounded shape of the liver cell nuclei, contrasting to the flattened endothelial cell nuclei. H and E. x660.

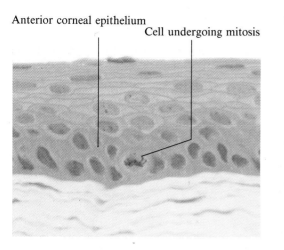

Anterior corneal epithelium
Cell undergoing mitosis

Metaphase chromosomes
Centromere   Acrocentric
    Metacentric   Arms   Submetacentric

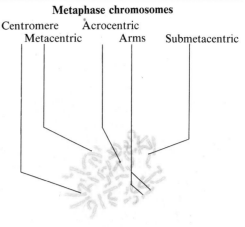

Fig. 1-21. Part of the **anterior corneal epithelium.** The characteristic appearance in histological sections of a cell undergoing mitotic division is seen in the basal part of the epithelium. H and E. x660.

Fig. 1-22. Normal human **metaphase chromosomes** in cells in which mitosis was arrested in metaphase by the addition of colchicine after three days of cultivation. Orcein staining. x660.

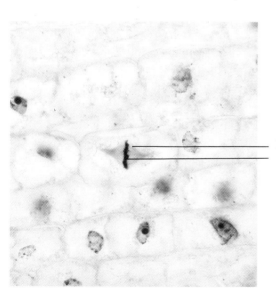

— Mitotic spindle
Metaphase plate of chromosomes

Fig. 1-23. Cells from the tip of the root of a bean seedling. The cell situated in the center of the picture shows a typical **mitotic spindle** and **metaphase plate.** Iron hematoxylin. x660.

Prophase

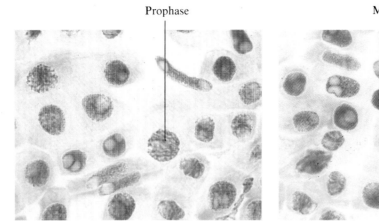

Metaphase

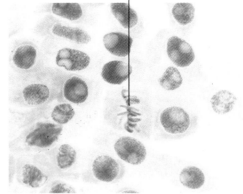

Fig. 1-24. Cells from the tip of the root of an onion seedling showing a cell in **prophase of mitosis.** The chromosomes are stained red using the Feulgen method which is specific to DNA (the cytoplasm is counterstained with Light Green). x660.

Fig. 1-25. Cells from the tip of the root of an onion seedling showing a cell in **metaphase.** Feulgen + Light Green. x660.

Anaphase   Telophase

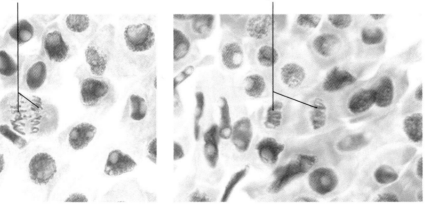

Fig. 1-26. Cells from the tip of the root of an onion seedling showing a cell in **anaphase.** Feulgen + Light Green. x660.

Fig. 1-27. Cells from the tip of the root of an onion seedling showing a cell in **telophase.** Feulgen + Light Green. x660.

CHAPTER 2

Epithelium

Semicircular duct   Simple squamous epithelium

Thyroid follicles   Simple cuboidal epithelium

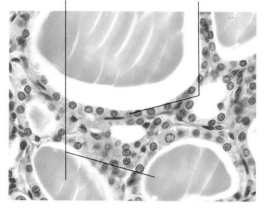

Fig. 2-1. Simple squamous epithelium lining **semi-circular duct of the internal ear.** H and E. x440.

Fig. 2-2. Simple cuboidal epithelium lining **thyroid follicles.** H and E. x440.

Simple columnar epithelium   Gastric mucosa

Simple columnar epithelium

Ductulus efferens   Cilia

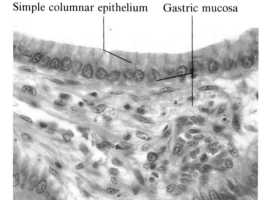

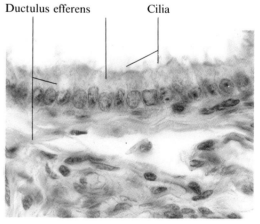

Fig. 2-3. Simple columnar epithelium of the **mucosa of the stomach.** H and E. x440.

Fig. 2-4. Simple columnar epithelium of the **ductuli efferentes of the epididymis.** Most of the cells have cilia on their luminal surface. Iron hematoxylin. x540.

Small   Simple columnar epithelium
intestinal mucosa   Brush border

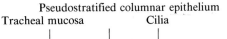

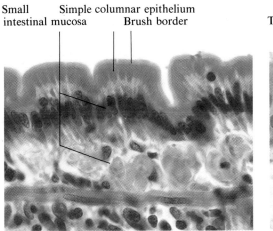

Fig. 2-5. Simple columnar epithelium of the **small intestinal mucosa.** Note the prominent luminal brush border. H and E. x660.

Pseudostratified columnar epithelium
Tracheal mucosa   Cilia

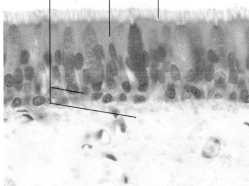

Fig. 2-6. Ciliated pseudostratified columnar epithelium of the **tracheal mucosa.** H and E. x540.

Pseudostratified columnar epithelium
Terminal bars   Ductus epididymidis

Stereocilia

Fig. 2-7. Pseudostratified columnar epithelium of the **ductus epididymidis.** The luminal surface of the cells has long stereocilia which form small tufts. Iron hematoxylin. x440.

Stratified
squamous epithelium Corneal stroma

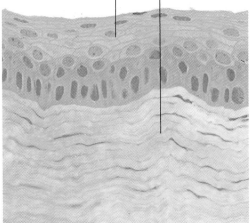

Fig. 2-8. Nonkeratinized stratified squamous epithelium of the **cornea** (anterior corneal epithelium). H and E. x440.

Stratified squamous epithelium   Esophageal mucosa

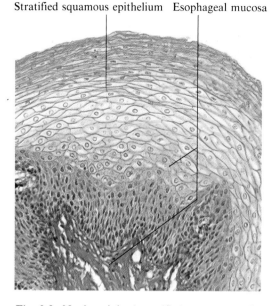

Keratinized stratified squamous epithelium
Epidermis   Dermal papillae

Horny layer

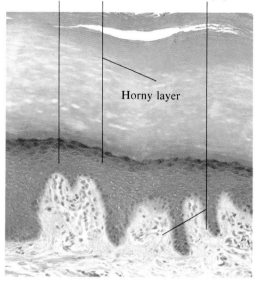

Fig. 2-9. Nonkeratinized stratified squamous epithelium of the **esophagus.** Note the much greater thickness of this epithelium compared with the anterior corneal epithelium (see Fig. 2-8). Van Gieson. x165.

Fig. 2-10. Keratinized stratified squamous epithelium of the **epidermis.** Note the thick horny layer. H and E. x135.

Stratified   Excretory duct
columnar epithelium   of submandibular gland

Mucosa of
urinary bladder   Transitional epithelium

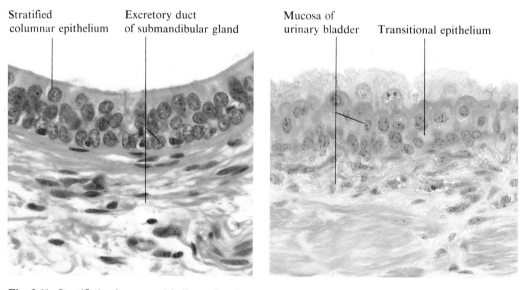

Fig. 2-11. Stratified columnar epithelium of an interlobular **excretory duct of the submandibular gland.** H and E. x540.

Fig. 2-12. Transitional epithelium of the **mucosa of the urinary bladder.** H and E. x440.

CHAPTER 3
Glands

Secretory granules   Pancreatic acini

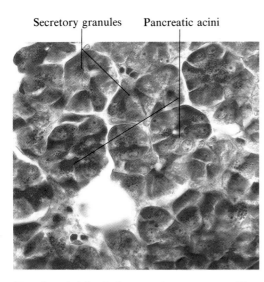

Fig. 3-1. Acini of the **exocrine pancreas.** The acinar cells contain red stained secretory granules and the secretory mechanism is merocrine (exocytotic). Liisberg's trichrome method. x440.

Apocrine sweat gland   Secretory cells

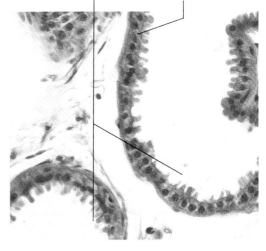

Fig. 3-2. Part of the secretory portion of an **apocrine sweat gland from the axilla.** Note the characteristic protrusions of the luminal surface of the secretory cells. These protrusions are (to some extent) pinched off by the apocrine secretory mechanism of these cells. H and E. x275.

Sebaceous gland   Hair in hair follicle

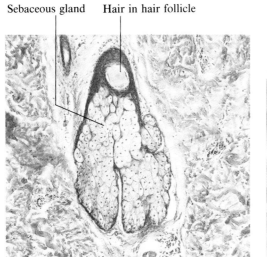

Fig. 3-3. Sebaceous gland of the skin. This is the only example in the human body of a gland secreting by a holocrine mechanism. H and E. x65.

Intestinal mucosa   Mucus   Goblet cells

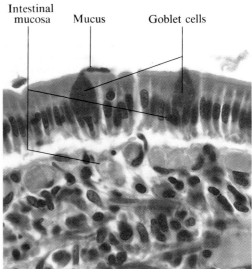

Fig. 3-4. Goblet cells of the **small intestinal mucosa.** The goblet cell to the left is in the process of emptying its content of mucin which is seen to float along the luminal surface of the epithelium. H and E. x660.

Goblet cells Small intestinal mucosa

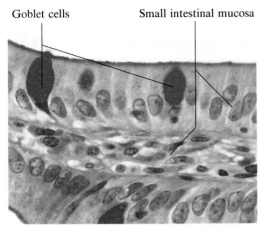

Fig. 3-5. Goblet cells of the **small intestinal mucosa.** The mucin is a glycoprotein and in this section has been stained specifically using the **PAS** reaction. PAS + H and E. x660.

Secretory epithelial sheath Gastric mucosa

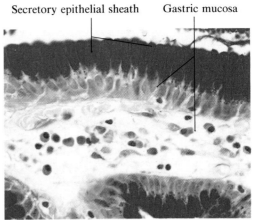

Fig. 3-6. Surface epithelium of the **gastric mucosa.** The section is stained using the PAS reaction and all the cells of the gastric surface epithelium are seen to be secretory, constituting the only example in the human body of a secretory epithelial sheath. PAS + Van Gieson. x440.

Intraepithelial glands of Littré Urethral mucosa

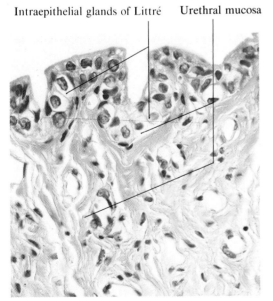

Fig. 3-7. Part of the mucosa of the **female urethra,** containing intraepithelial glands of Littré. H and E. x440.

Large intestinal mucosa Simple tubular glands (crypts of Lieberkühn)

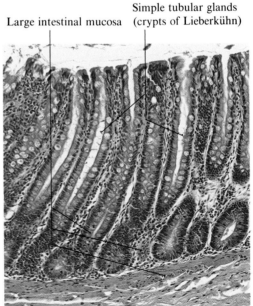

Fig. 3-8. Simple tubular glands (crypts of Lieberkühn) of the **large intestinal mucosa.** H and E. x110.

Acini   Exocrine pancreas

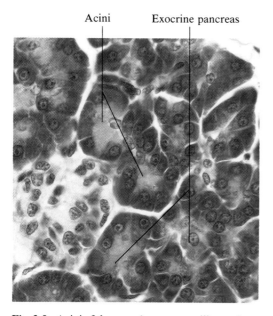

Fig. 3-9. Acini of the **exocrine pancreas** illustrating the appearance of acinar secretory portions. H and E. x540.

Alveoli   Prostate

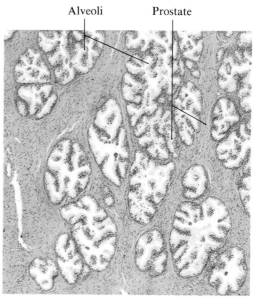

Fig. 3-10. Alveoli of the **prostate** illustrating the appearance of alveolar secretory portions. Van Gieson. x45.

Mixed salivary gland of tongue
Mucous acini   Serous acini

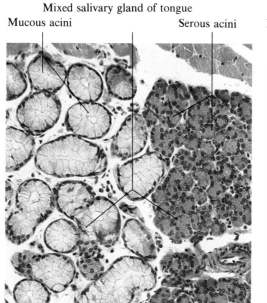

Fig. 3-11. Mucous and serous secretory portions (acini) of **salivary gland of the tongue.** H and E. x165.

Submandibular gland
Demilunes   Mixed secretory portions

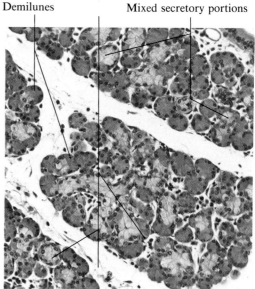

Fig. 3-12. Part of the **submandibular gland** showing numerous mixed (seromucous) secretory portions, in many of which the serous cells form demilunes of Von Ebner. H and E. x165.

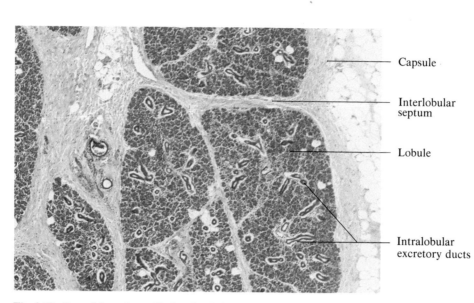

Capsule

Interlobular
septum

Lobule

Intralobular
excretory ducts

Fig. 3-13. Part of the **submandibular gland** showing the general histological structure of an exocrine gland. Part of a lobe is seen (situated immediately beneath the capsule) and the subdivision of the lobe into lobules by connective tissue septa is apparent. H and E. x40.

Salivary
(striated) duct   Intercalated duct

Interlobular
excretory duct   Intralobular salivary ducts

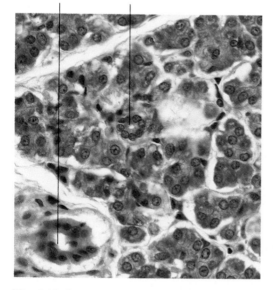

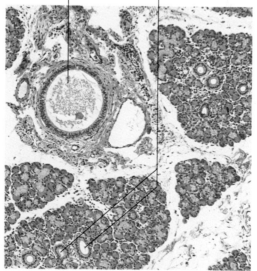

Fig. 3-14. Part of the **parotid gland** showing an intercalated duct and a salivary (striated duct), both of which are intralobular. H and E. x440.

Fig. 3-15. Part of the **submandibular gland** showing an interlobular excretory duct and numerous intralobular (salivary) ducts. H and E. x65.

Secretory cells — Hormone-containing secretory granules — Capillary

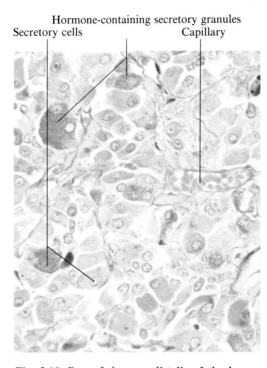

Secretory cells — Thyroid follicles — Secretory product

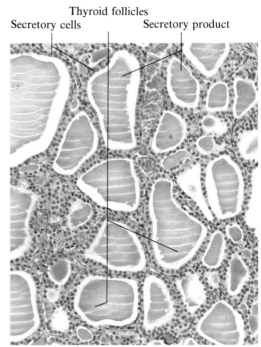

Fig. 3-16. Part of the **pars distalis of the hypophysis.** This is a characteristic example of an endocrine gland. The secretory product (hormone) is stored in intracellular secretory granules. The secretory cells are arranged in cords or clumps. PAS + orange G. x440.

Fig. 3-17. Part of the **thyroid gland.** This is the only example in the human body of an endocrine gland storing its secretory product extracellularly (in the lumen of the thyroid follicles) and having the secretory cells arranged in the form of follicles. H and E. x165.

CHAPTER 4

Connective Tissue Proper

Bundles of collagenous fibers

Collagenous fibers

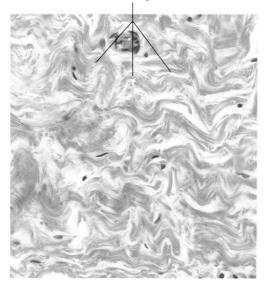

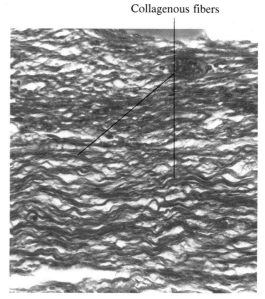

Fig. 4-1. Dense, irregular connective tissue of the **mammary gland** showing typical wavy bundles of collagenous fibers. H and E. x275.

Fig. 4-2. Dense, irregular connective tissue of the **tunica albuginea of the ovary.** The collagenous fibers stain intensely blue with the aniline blue used in this trichrome staining. Azan. x275.

Collagenous fibers

Reticular fibers

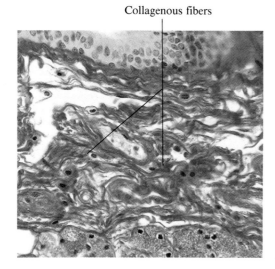

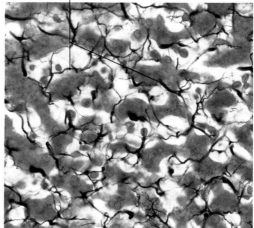

Fig. 4-3. Part of connective tissue septum in the **parotid gland** showing red stained collagenous fibers. Van Gieson. x275.

Fig. 4-4. Silver impregnated reticular fibers within **lobule of the liver.** Note that the reticular fibers branch and anastomose frequently, forming a reticulum (hence their name). Bielschowsky. x275.

Basement membrane   Tubules of kidney

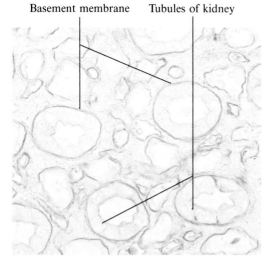

Fig. 4-5. Basement membranes of **tubules of the kidney,** stained red using the PAS reaction. x340.

Elastic fibers   Dermal connective tissue

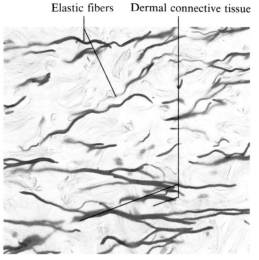

Fig. 4-6. Elastic fibers of the **dermis of the skin,** stained selectively with orcein. x275.

Internal   Wall of muscular artery
elastic lamina   Elastic fibers

Fibroblasts   Bundles of
                                    collagenous fibers

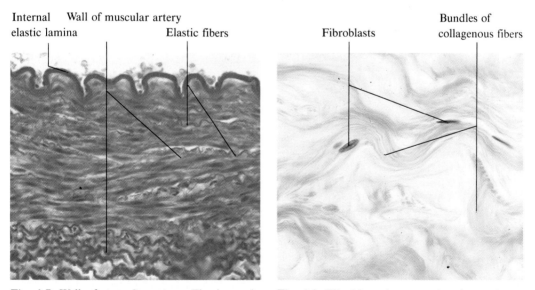

Fig. 4-7. Wall of **muscular artery.** The internal elastic lamina (which is an elastic membrane) and the elastic fibers are stained selectively with orcein. x275.

Fig. 4-8. Fibroblasts in connective tissue of the **mammary gland.** Note that only the nuclei of the fibroblasts are seen distinctly. H and E. x440.

Mesenchymal cells   Mesenchyme

Reticular cells   Cellular reticulum

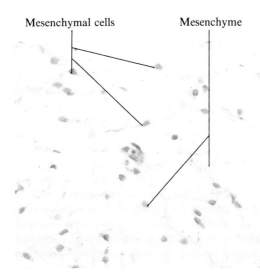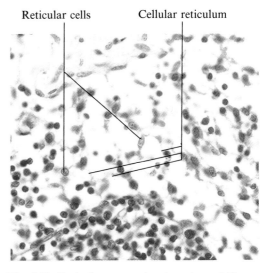

Fig. 4-9. Primitive connective tissue – **mesenchyme** – of a fetus. Note the very loose character of the tissue and the stellate appearance of the mesenchymal cells. H and E. x275.

Fig. 4-10. Reticular connective tissue in **medullary sinus of a lymph node.** The reticular fibres are not stained and only the reticular cells, forming a cellular reticulum, are seen. H and E. x440.

Unilocular adipose cells
Cytoplasmic rim   Nucleus

Unilocular adipose cells

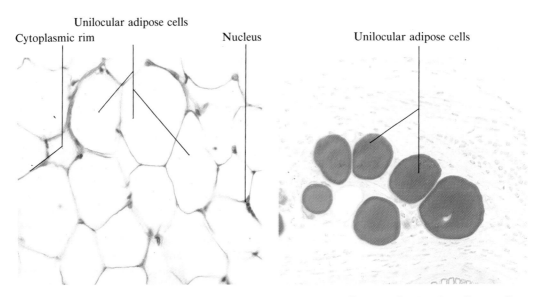

Fig. 4-11. Ordinary (white) adipose tissue consisting of unilocular adipose cells. The lipid has been dissolved during the preparatory procedures and the cells appear empty with only a thin rim of cytoplasm. H and E. x275.

Fig. 4-12. Small group of **unilocular adipose cells.** The lipid has been preserved by fixation and staining with osmium. x165.

Multilocular adipose cells   Brown adipose tissue

Alveolar
macrophage (dust cell)   Small bronchiole

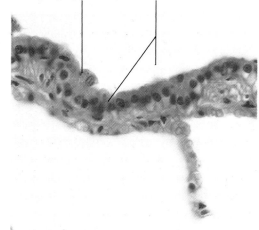

Fig. 4-13. Brown adipose tissue from interscapular region of a rat, consisting of multilocular adipose cells. H and E. x440.

Fig. 4-14. Alveolar macrophage lying on the surface of the epithelium of a small **bronchiole.** The macrophage contains engulfed coal dust particles and is often termed a »dust cell«. H and E. x440.

Macrophages containing lithium carmine

Eosinophilic granulocytes
Plasma cell   Fibroblast

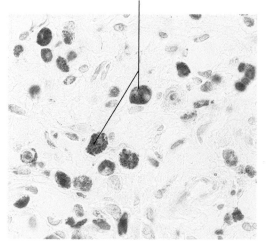

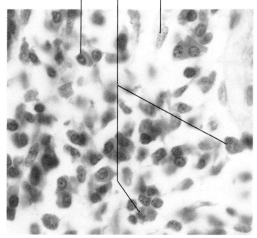

Fig. 4-15. Macrophages in loose connective tissue, stained supravitally by the addition of lithium carmine to a preparation of living tissue. The red lithium carmine particles have been phagocytosed by the macrophages. x440.

Fig. 4-16. Part of the **lamina propria of the small intestine** which is a very cell-rich loose connective tissue. H and E. x660.

Mast cells

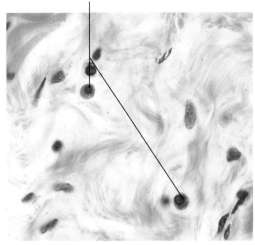

Mast cells

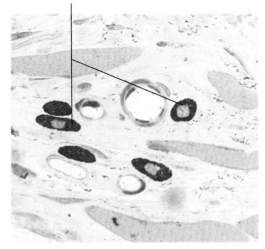

Fig. 4-17. Mast cells in dense connective tissue of the **mammary gland.** H and E. x540.

Fig. 4-18. Mast cells in connective tissue of the **tongue.** The acid glycosaminoglycan (heparin), contained in the cytoplasmic granules, stains metachromatically with toluidine blue in this section. x660.

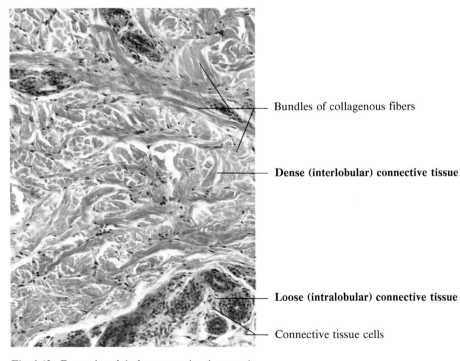

Bundles of collagenous fibers

Dense (interlobular) connective tissue

Loose (intralobular) connective tissue

Connective tissue cells

Fig. 4-19. Dense, interlobular connective tissue and loose intralobular connective tissue of the **mammary gland.** H and E. x110.

Tendon   Bundles of collagenous fibers

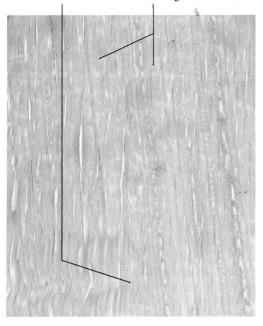

Fig. 4-20. Longitudinal section through a **tendon,** an example of dense regular connective tissue. H and E. x110.

Bundles of collagenous fibers
Tendon   Cells

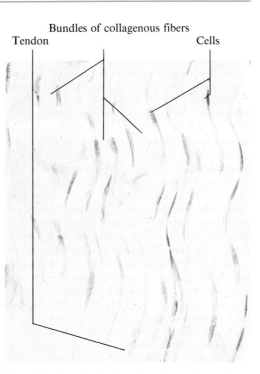

Fig. 4-21. Longitudinal section through a **tendon,** seen at higher magnification. Note the almost rectangular cells, with flattened nuclei, forming parallel rows between the bundles of collagenous fibers. H and E. x440.

Mucous connective tissue (Wharton's jelly)
Intercellular substance   Cells

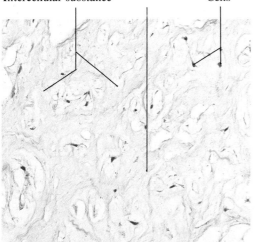

Fig. 4-22. Mucous connective tissue (Wharton's jelly) of the **umbilical cord.** Note the very abundant intercellular substance. H and E. x135.

Reticular
connective tissue   Reticular fibers

Fig. 4-23. Reticular connective tissue of a **lymph node.** The reticular fibers are stained by silver impregnation. Bielschowsky. x275.

CHAPTER 5

Blood and Bone Marrow

Lumen of small artery   Erythrocytes

Erythrocytes   Blood platelets

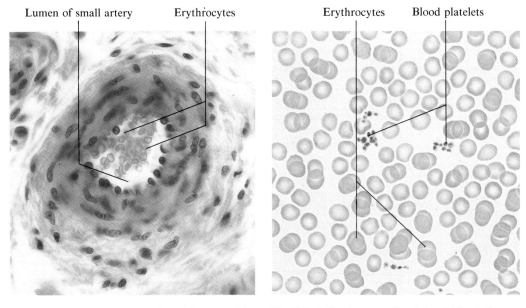

Fig. 5-1. Cross-sectional view of a small artery with erythrocytes in the lumen, showing the general appearance of **erythrocytes in tissue sections.** H and E. x440.

Fig. 5-2. Stained smear of peripheral blood, showing **erythrocytes** and clumps of **blood platelets.** May-Grünwald-Giemsa staining. x660.

Neutrophilic granulocyte

Eosinophilic granulocyte

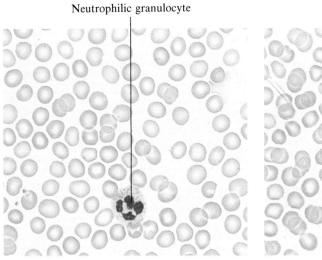

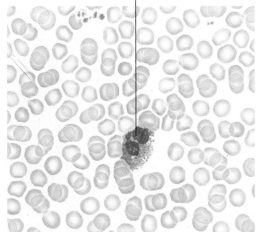

Fig. 5-3. Stained smear of peripheral blood showing **neutrophilic granulocyte.** May-Grünwald-Giemsa. x660.

Fig. 5-4. Stained smear of peripheral blood showing **eosinophilic granulocyte.** Note the characteristic two-lobed nucleus with a small intermediate chromatin clump. May-Grünwald-Giemsa. x660.

Basophilic granulocyte

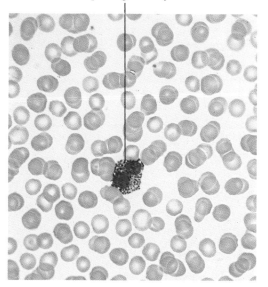

Lymphocytes Neutrophilic granulocyte

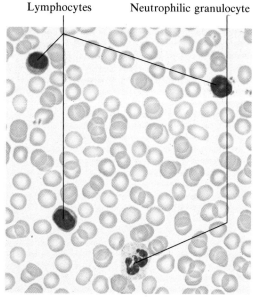

Fig. 5-5. Stained smear of peripheral blood showing **basophilic granulocyte.** May-Grünwald-Giemsa. x660.

Fig. 5-6. Stained smear of peripheral blood, showing three **lymphocytes** and a **neutrophilic granulocyte.** May-Grünwald-Giemsa. x660.

Monocyte

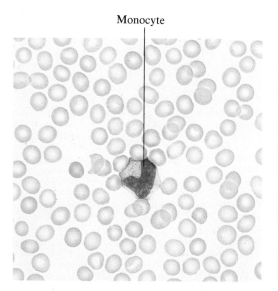

Neutrophilic granulocyte Eosinophilic granulocyte

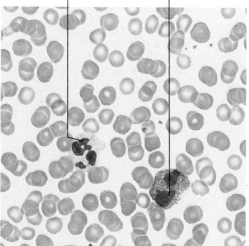

Fig. 5-7. Stained smear of peripheral blood showing **monocyte.** Note the characteristic folding of the peripheral cytoplasm. May-Grünwald-Giemsa. x660.

Fig. 5-8. Stained smear of peripheral blood, showing **neutrophilic granulocyte** and **eosinophilic granulocyte.** Note the pronounced lobation of the neutrophilic granulocyte. May-Grünwald-Giemsa. x660.

Fetal hepatic tissue   Megakaryocytes

Fetal (primitive) bone marrow   Bone tissue

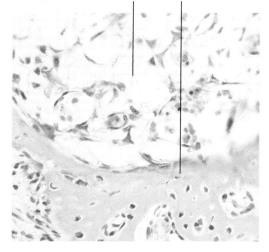

Fig. 5-9. Section of human fetus in third fetal month, showing **hemopoiesis in the liver.** H and E. x275.

Fig. 5-10. Primitive bone marrow from a human fetus in third fetal month. Note the nucleate erythrocytes in some of the newly formed blood vessels. H and E. x275.

Hemopoietically active (red) bone marrow
Hemopoietic compartment   Sinusoids

Reticulocytes

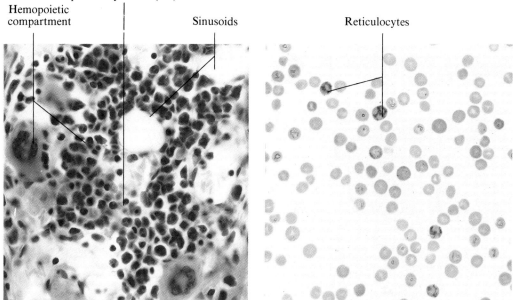

Fig. 5-11. Part of **hemopoietically active (red) bone marrow.** Note the two megakaryocytes. H and E. x440.

Fig. 5-12. Smear of peripheral blood, stained supravitally with brilliant cresyl blue for the demonstration of **reticulocytes.** The blood is obtained from a patient with an increased number of reticulocytes in the blood. x660.

Basophilic erythoblast
Myelocyte Stem cell

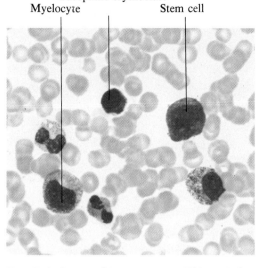

Promyelocyte Myelocyte

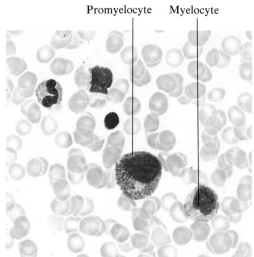

Fig. 5-13. Smear of bone marrow. This and the following stained smears of bone marrow illustrate various stages of hemopoiesis and have been obtained by bone marrow aspiration. May-Grünwald-Giemsa. x660.

Fig. 5-14. Smear of bone marrow. May-Grünwald-Giemsa. x660.

Metamyelocyte (bandform) Myelocytes

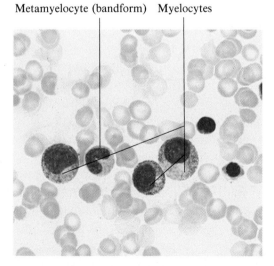

Polychromatophilic
erythroblasts Normoblast

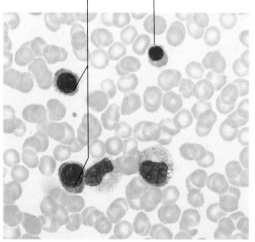

Fig. 5-15. Smear of bone marrow. May-Grünwald-Giemsa. x660.

Fig. 5-16. Smear of bone marrow. May-Grünwald-Giemsa. x660.

Normoblasts

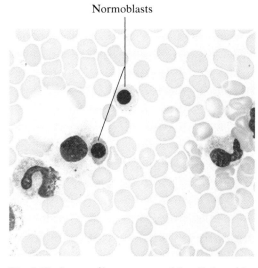

Metaphase plate

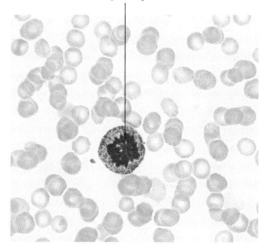

Fig. 5-17. Smear of bone marrow. May-Grünwald-Giemsa. x660.

Fig. 5-18. Smear of bone marrow, showing a cell in metaphase of mitotic division. May-Grünwald-Giemsa. x660.

Megakaryoblast

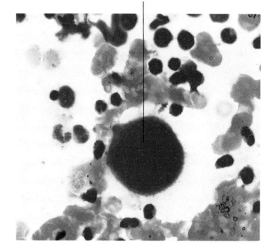

Megakaryocyte

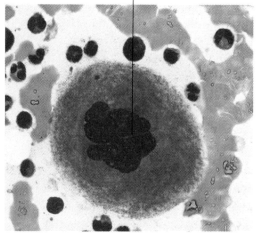

Fig. 5-19. Smear of bone marrow showing a **megakaryoblast.** May-Grünwald-Giemsa. x660.

Fig. 5-20. Smear of bone marrow showing a **megakaryocyte.** Note the lobation of the nucleus. May–Grünwald–Giemsa. x600.

CHAPTER 6

The Skeletal Tissues

Perichrondrium   Embryonic cartilage   Chondroblast   Chondrocytes   Embryonic cartilage

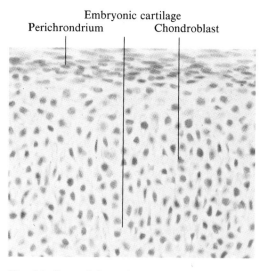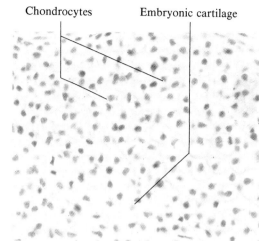

Fig. 6-1. Part of the **embryonic cartilage** from a fetus in the third fetal month. Note the densely packed chondroblasts with almost no intervening cartilage matrix. H and E. x340.

Fig. 6-2. Part of **embryonic cartilage** from the same fetus as Fig. 6-1, but at a slightly later stage of development. The chondroblasts have now developed into chondrocytes. These are less densely packed than the chondroblasts because of the presence of more abundant cartilage matrix which they secrete. H and E. x340.

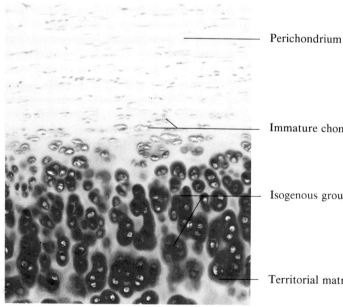

Perichondrium

Immature chondrocytes

Isogenous groups

Territorial matrix (capsule)

Fig. 6-3. Superficial part of **tracheal cartilage,** showing the appearance of mature hyaline cartilage. H and E. x135.

Elastic cartilage
Chondrocytes   Elastic fibers

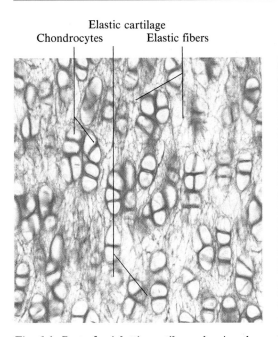

Fibrous cartilage
Chondrocytes   Collagenous fibers

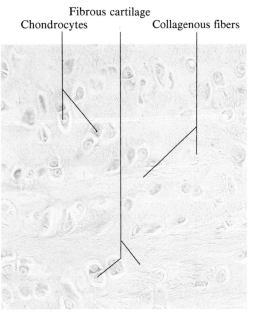

Fig. 6-4. Part of **epiglottic cartilage,** showing the appearance of elastic cartilage. Orcein staining. x165.

Fig. 6-5. Fibrous cartilage from the articular surface of a vertebra. H and E. x275.

Haversian system (osteon)
Osteocytes in lacunae   Lamellae

Haversian system (osteon)
Osteocytes in lacunae   Lamellae

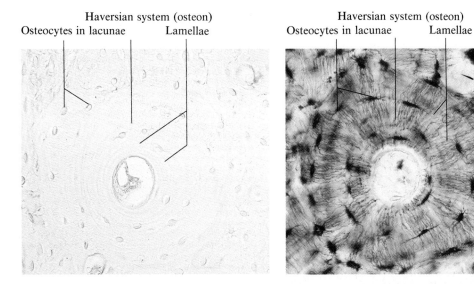

Fig. 6-6. Section of decalcified **compact bone,** showing a Haversian system (osteon). Eosin staining. x275.

Fig. 6-7. Ground section of **compact bone,** showing a Haversian system (osteon). x235.

Canaliculi   Interstitial lamellae   Haversian canal   Lamellae   Haversian systems (osteons)   Lacunae

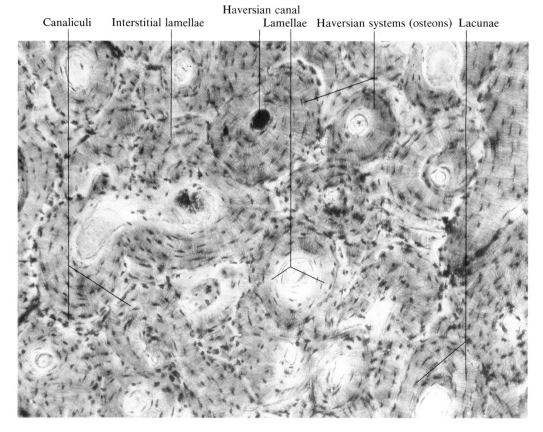

Fig. 6-8. Ground section of **compact bone,** showing numerous Haversian systems and interstitial lamellae. x110.

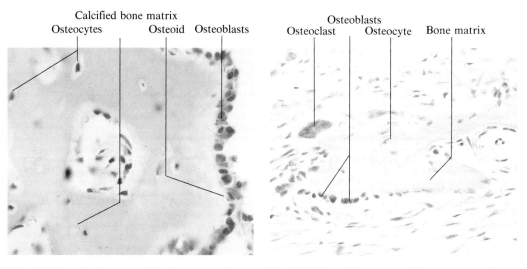

Calcified bone matrix
Osteocytes   Osteoid   Osteoblasts

Osteoblasts
Osteoclast   Osteocyte   Bone matrix

Fig. 6-9. Part of **primary ossification center** from the primordium of a flat bone of the vault (from a human fetus in third fetal month). H and E. x440.

Fig. 6-10. Part of **primary ossification center** from the primordium of a flat bone of the vault (from a human fetus in third fetal month). A small trabecula of newly formed bone is seen. H and E. x275.

Primitive cancellous bone   Vascular
Trabeculae of bone   connective tissue

Primitive compact bone
Bone   Vascular connective tissue

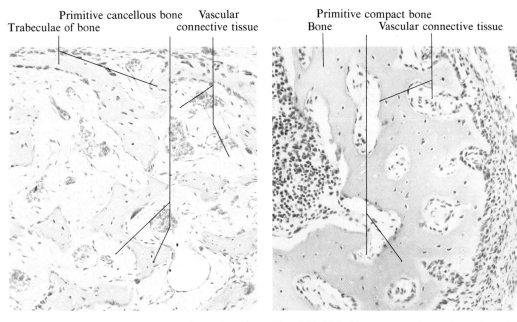

Fig. 6-11. Primitive cancellous bone from the primordium of a flat bone of the vault (from a human fetus in third fetal month). H and E. x135.

Fig. 6-12. Primitive compact bone from the primordium of a flat bone of the vault (from a human fetus in third fetal month). H and E. x165.

Primary (diaphyseal) ossification center
Perichondrium   Hypertrophic chondrocytes

Primary (diaphyseal) ossification center
Calcified cartilage matrix | Hypertrophic chondrocytes

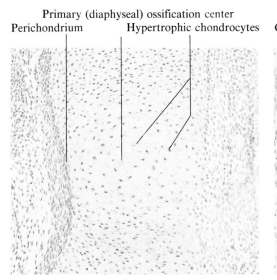

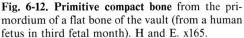

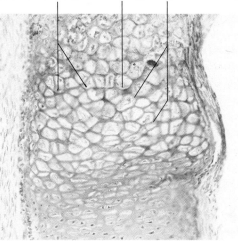

Fig. 6-13. Primary (diaphyseal) ossification center formed in the hyaline cartilage model of a long bone during endochondral osteogenesis. H and E. x110.

Fig. 6-14. Primary (diaphyseal) ossification center at a slightly later stage of development, showing calcification of the cartilage matrix. H and E. x110.

Diaphyseal
ossification center   Periosteal collar

Periosteal bud
Calcified cartilage matrix   Periosteal collar

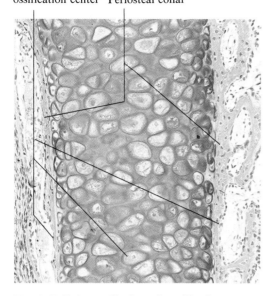

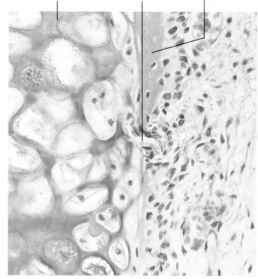

Fig. 6-15. Primary (diaphyseal) ossification center from the endochondral primordium of a long bone (from a human fetus in third fetal month). The cartilage model is now seen to be surrounded by the periosteal collar which consists of bone. H and E. x110.

Fig. 6-16. Part of **primary ossification center** from the endochondral development of a long bone (from a human fetus in third fetal month). A periosteal bud has now penetrated the periosteal collar. H and E. x275.

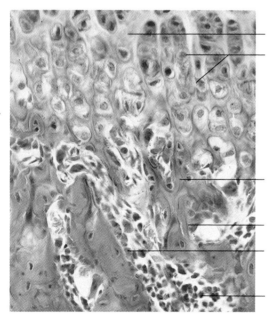

— Calcified cartilage matrix

— Hypertrophic chondrocytes in lacunae

— Calcified cartilage matrix

— Newly formed bone

— Layer of osteoblasts

— Primitive bone marrow

Fig. 6-17. Endochondral ossification in a long bone (from a human fetus in third fetal month). Note the trabeculae of calcified cartilage matrix (stained blue), surrounded by a layer of newly formed eosinophilic bone (stained red). H and E. x275.

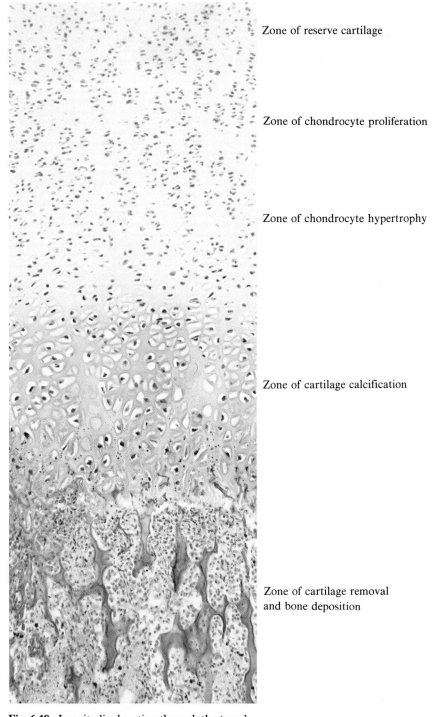

Zone of reserve cartilage

Zone of chondrocyte proliferation

Zone of chondrocyte hypertrophy

Zone of cartilage calcification

Zone of cartilage removal
and bone deposition

Fig. 6-18. Longitudinal section through the **transition between the diaphysis and epiphysis** in a long bone, in which growth in length takes place by endochondral ossification. H and E. x110.

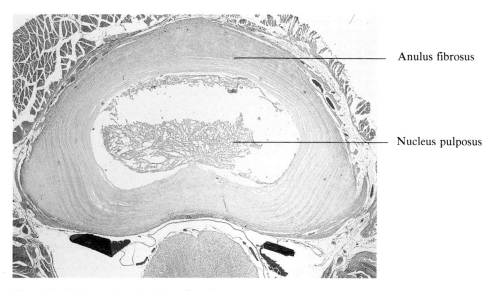

Anulus fibrosus

Nucleus pulposus

Fig. 6-19. Horizontal section through an **intervertebral disk.** H and E. x10.

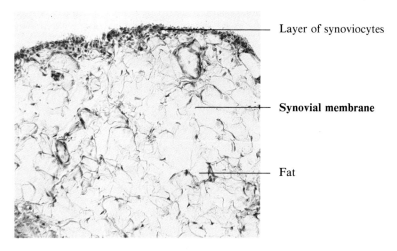

Layer of synoviocytes

Synovial membrane

Fat

Fig. 6-20. Part of **synovial membrane** of adipose type (the surface layer of synoviocytes is separated from the fibrous capsule by a layer of fat). H and E. x135.

CHAPTER 7

Muscular Tissue

Nuclei   Smooth muscle fibers

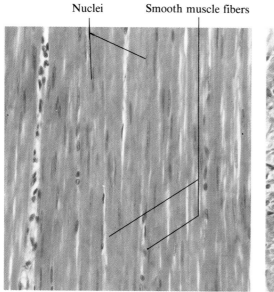

Nuclei   Smooth muscle fibers

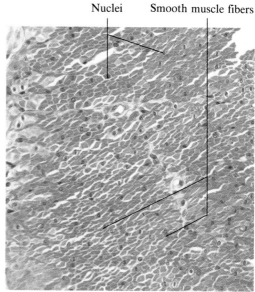

Fig. 7-1. Longitudinal section through smooth muscle cells in the wall of the **large intestine.** Note the very long nuclei situated in the central part of the smooth muscle fibers. H and E. x275.

Fig. 7-2. Transverse section through smooth muscle cells in the wall of the **large intestine.** H and E. x275.

Nuclei   Skeletal muscle fibers

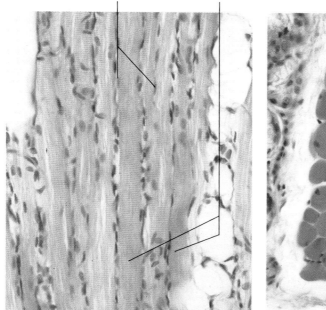

Nuclei   Skeletal muscle fibers

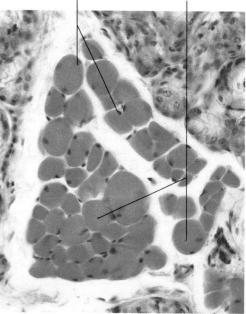

Fig. 7-3. Longitudinal section through skeletal muscle fibers of the **tongue.** Note the cross-striation and the peripherally situated nuclei. H and E. x275.

Fig. 7-4. Transverse section through skeletal muscle fibers of the **tongue.** H and E. x275.

Cardiac muscle fibers   Nuclei   Cardiac muscle fibers   Nuclei

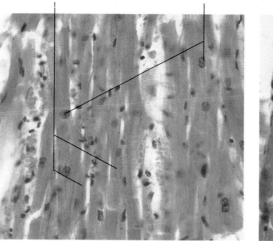 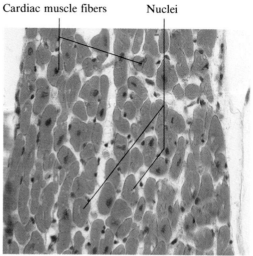

Fig. 7-5. Longitudinal section through **cardiac muscle fibers.** Note the inconspicuous cross-striation and the centrally situated nuclei. H and E. x275.

Fig. 7-6. Transverse section through **cardiac muscle fibers.** H and E. x275.

Smooth muscle fibers   Nuclei   Smooth muscle fibers   Nuclei

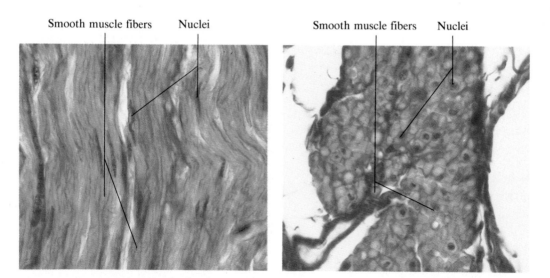

Fig. 7-7. Longitudinal section through smooth muscle fibers in the wall of the **esophagus.** Van Gieson. x540.

Fig. 7-8. Transverse section through smooth muscle fibers in the wall of the **esophagus.** Van Gieson. x540.

A band   I band   Myofibrils   Z line   H band

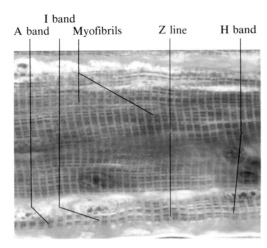

Fig. 7-9. Longitudinal section through **skeletal muscle.** Most of the picture is occupied by a single muscle fiber, which is seen to consist of several myofibrils. Azan. x880.

A band   I band   Myofibrils   Z line   H band   Capillary

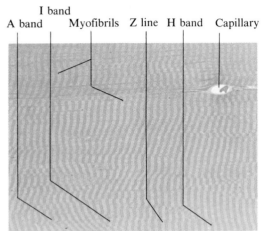

Fig. 7-10. Longitudinal section through **skeletal muscle.** Part of two muscle fibers are seen, separated by a narrow endomysium, in which a capillary is seen. Epon-embedded section, stained with methylene blue. x640.

Tendon   Skeletal muscle fibers   Cardiac muscle cell   Intercalated disks

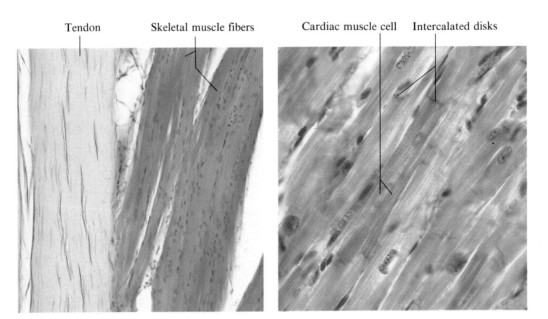

Fig. 7-11. Longitudinal section through the **transition between skeletal muscle fibers and their associated tendon.** H and E. x135.

Fig. 7-12. Longitudinal section through **cardiac muscle.** Note the step-like appearance of the intercalated disks. Azan. x440.

Cardiac muscle fibers   Capillaries   Capillaries   Skeletal muscle fibers

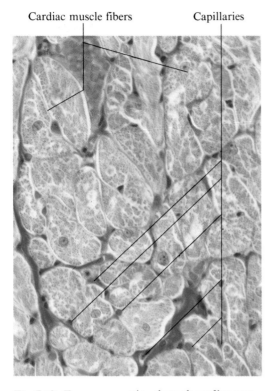 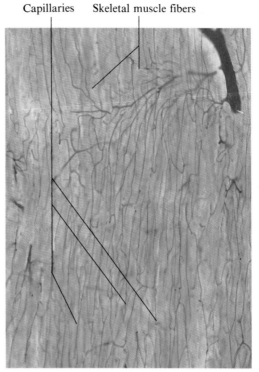

Fig. 7-13. Transverse section through **cardiac muscle,** showing the abundance of capillaries between the cardiac muscle fibers. Azan. x440.

Fig. 7-14. Preparation of **skeletal muscle,** where the microvasculature has been demonstrated by the injection of lithium carmine into the arterial blood stream. x135.

CHAPTER 8

Nervous Tissue

Soma
(cell body)   Dendrites   Spinae   Axon

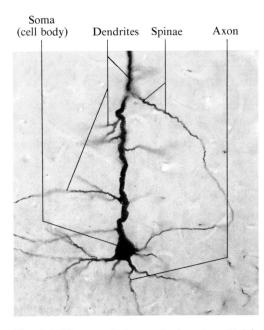

Fig. 8-1. Neuron of the **cerebral cortex.** Golgi method. x275.

Pyramidal cells

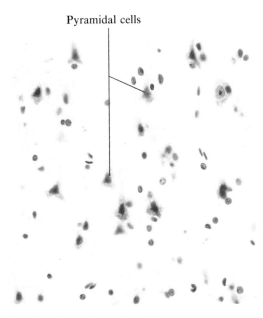

Fig. 8–2. Pyramidal cells of the **cerebral cortex.** Toluidine blue. x275.

Dendritic tree   Purkinje cell

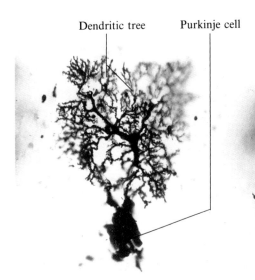

Fig. 8-3. Purkinje cell of the **cerebellar cortex.** Note the extensively branched dendritic tree. Golgi method. x275.

Motor neuron from anterior horn
Dendrites   Axon   Soma

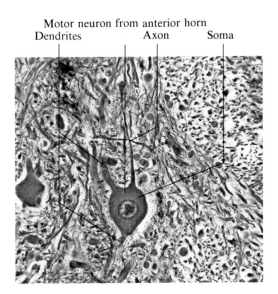

Fig. 8-4. Motor neuron of the **anterior horn of the spinal cord.** Bodian staining. x275.

Motor neuron from anterior horn
Nissl bodies

Sensory neuron from spinal ganglion
Nissl bodies

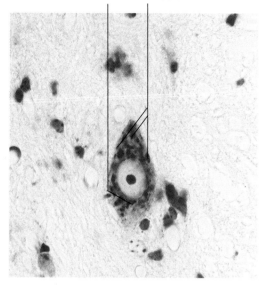

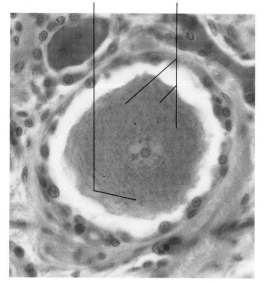

Fig. 8-5. Motor neuron from the **anterior horn of the spinal cord.** The Nissl pattern in this type of neuron is coarsely granular. Thionine staining. x540.

Fig. 8-6. Sensory neuron of a **spinal ganglion,** showing finely granular appearance of Nissl bodies. H and E. x440.

Neurofibrils

Boutons en passage

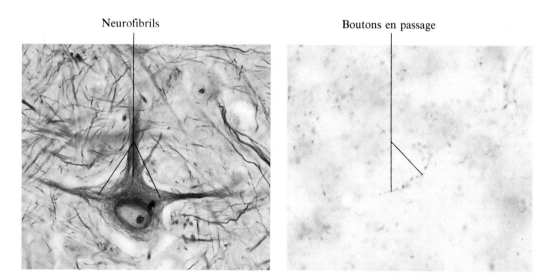

Fig. 8-7. Multipolar neuron of the **medulla oblongata.** Note the distinct neurofibrils in the cytoplasm. Cajal staining. x760.

Fig. 8-8. Immunohistochemical demonstration of enkephalin in axons of the periaqueductal gray substance of the **mesencephalon.** The axons show boutons en passage. x660.

Astrocytes   Perivascular foot processes

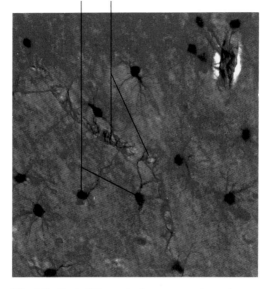

Microglia (glioblasts)

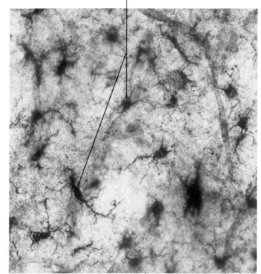

Fig. 8-9. Part of the central nervous system, showing **astroglia.** Note the characteristic perivascular foot processes. Cajal gold sublimate method. x375.

Fig. 8-10. Section of the central nervous system showing **microglia.** Timm sulfide silver staining. x375.

Oligodendrocytes   Ependyma

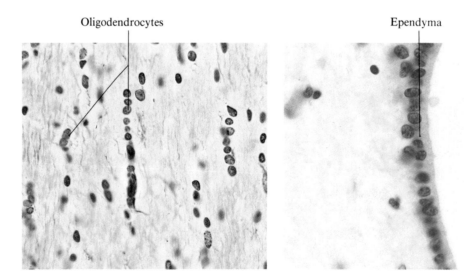

Fig. 8-11. Section through **white matter of the central nervous system** showing oligodendrocytes. The oligodendrocytes lie in rows between the nerve fibers and are of the so-called interfascicular type. Penfield staining. x375.

Fig. 8-12. Ependyma lining the **central canal of the medulla oblongata.** Toluidine blue. x660.

Nerve fibers   Myelin sheaths   Axons   Nerve fibers

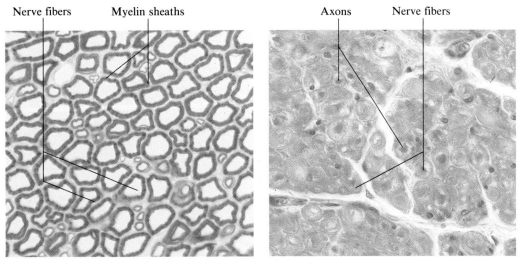

Fig. 8-13. Transverse section through **peripheral nerve.** The myelin sheaths are stained with osmium and are seen as black rings surrounding the unstained axons. Note the variation in size of the nerve fibers. x540.

Fig. 8-14. Transverse section through **peripheral nerve.** The section is stained with hematoxylin and eosin, and remnants of the myelin sheaths are seen as lightly stained rings surrounding the stained axons. x375.

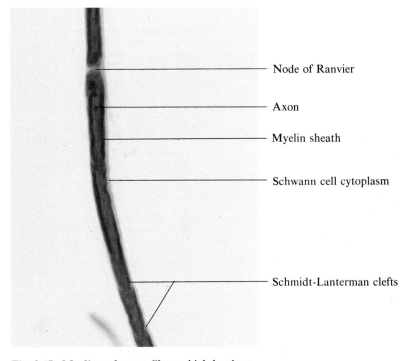

Node of Ranvier

Axon

Myelin sheath

Schwann cell cytoplasm

Schmidt-Lanterman clefts

Fig. 8-15. Myelinated nerve fiber, which has been isolated from an osmium-fixed preparation. x440.

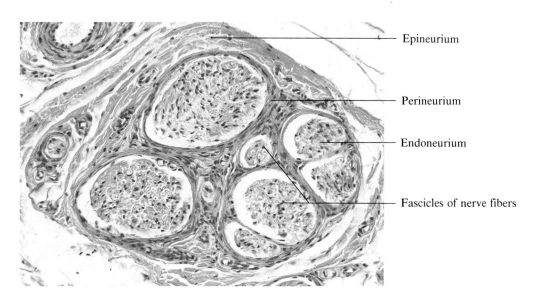

Epineurium

Perineurium

Endoneurium

Fascicles of nerve fibers

Fig. 8-16. Cross-sectional view of a **peripheral nerve,** illustrating the histological organization of the connective tissue component of peripheral nerves. H and E. x165.

Nerve fibers Schwann cell nuclei Perineurium

Capsule Spinal ganglion Ganglion cells

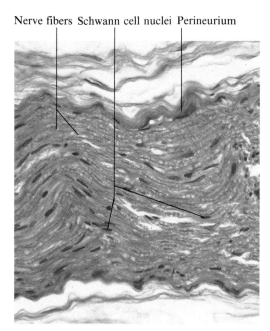

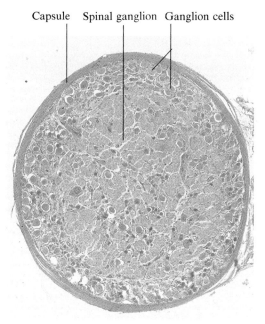

Fig. 8-17. Longitudinal section through small **peripheral nerve.** Note the characteristic wavy appearance. H and E. x275.

Fig. 8-18. Transected **spinal ganglion.** H and E. x27.

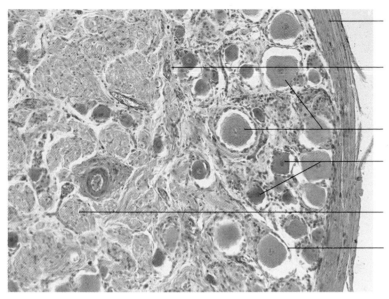

Connective tissue capsule

Vascular connective tissue

Nerve cell bodies (A cells)

Nerve cell bodies (B cells)

Bundle of nerve fibers

Layer of satellite cells

Fig. 8-19. Part of a **spinal ganglion.** Note the great variation in size of the nerve cell bodies. H and E. x110.

Connective tissue capsule   Layer of satellite cells
Nerve cell bodies   Nerve fibers

Nerve cell bodies   Fibroblasts

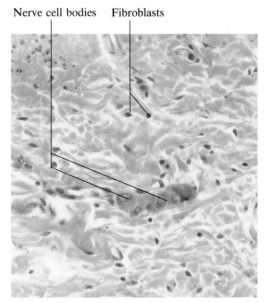

Fig. 8-20. Part of an **autonomic (sympathetic) ganglion.** Note the relatively uniform size of the nerve cell bodies which generally are smaller than those of spinal ganglia. (cp. Fig. 8-19). H and E. x110.

Fig. 8-21. Small intramural **autonomic (parasympathetic) ganglion** from the intestinal wall (from the plexus submucosus of Meissner). Note the large size of the nerve cell bodies compared to the fibroblasts in the surrounding connective tissue. H and E. x375.

Genital corpuscle

Nerve fiber   Capsule

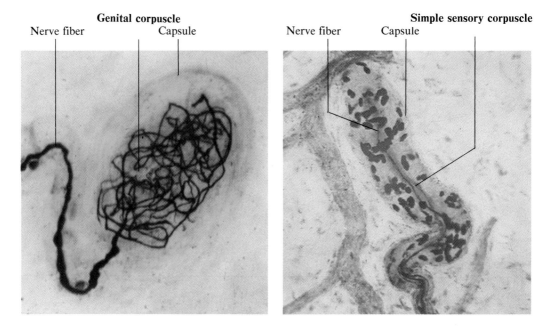

Fig. 8-22. Genital corpuscle from the **skin of the labium minus.** Bielschowski staining, Lavrentiev's modification. x345.

Simple sensory corpuscle

Nerve fiber   Capsule

Fig. 8-23. Simple sensory corpuscle from the **skin of the lip.** Bielschowski staining, Lavrentiev's modification. x960.

Corpuscle of Meissner

Nerve fiber   Capsule

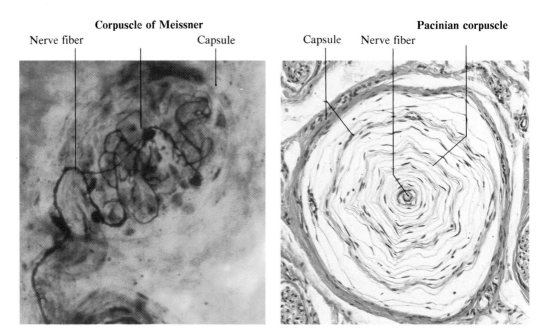

Fig. 8-24. Corpuscle of Meissner from the **skin of the labium minus.** Bielschowski staining, Lavrentiev's modification. x345.

Pacinian corpuscle

Capsule   Nerve fiber

Fig. 8-25. Pacinian corpuscle from the **skin of a finger.** H and E. x135.

Molecular layer   Granular layer

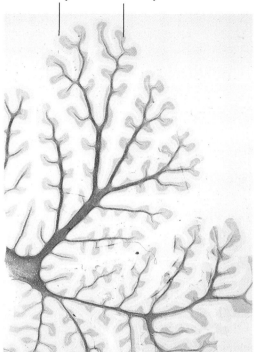

Molecular layer   Granular layer

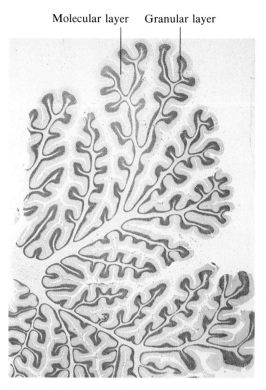

Fig. 8-26. Sagittal section through the **vermis of the cerebellum,** illustrating the intensive folding of the cerebellar cortex. Holzer staining. x3.

Fig. 8-27. Sagittal section through the **vermis of the cerebellum.** Toluidine blue. x3.

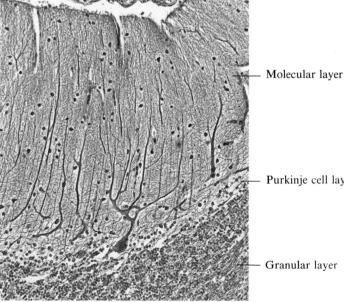

— Molecular layer

— Purkinje cell layer

— Granular layer

Fig. 8-28. Part of the **cerebellar cortex,** illustrating the general, three-layered structure. Cajal staining. x165.

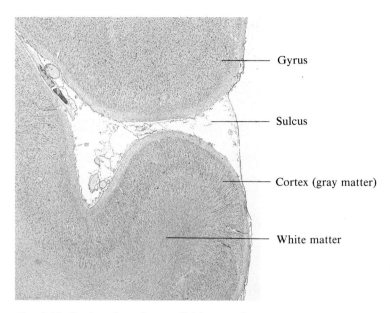

—— Gyrus

—— Sulcus

—— Cortex (gray matter)

—— White matter

Fig. 8-29. Section through superficial part of a **cerebral hemisphere,** showing the general appearance of the cerebral cortex and underlying white matter. Gallocyanin-chromallum. x10.

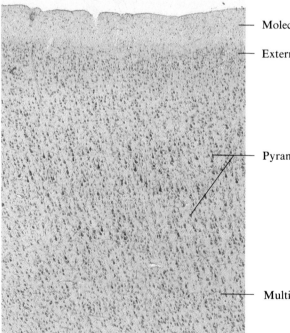

—— Molecular layer
—— External granular layer

—— Pyramidal cells

—— Multiform layer

Fig. 8-30. Part of the **cerebral cortex,** illustrating the general cytoarchitecture of the neocortex (isocortex) in which six layers usually can be distinguished. In this section, the boundaries between the third, fourth and fifth layers are not distinct. Toluidine blue. x40.

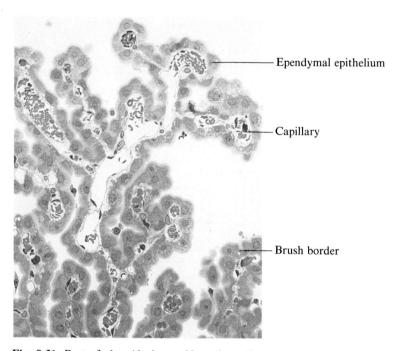

Ependymal epithelium

Capillary

Brush border

Fig. 8-31. Part of **choroid plexus.** Note the well developed brush border covering the luminal surface of the ependymal epithelial cells. Epon-embedded section stained with methylene blue. x275.

CHAPTER 9

The Circulatory System

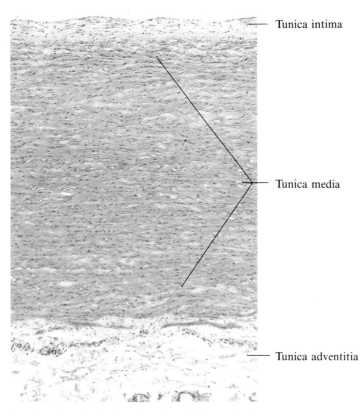

Tunica intima

Tunica media

Tunica adventitia

Fig. 9-1. Longitudinal section through the wall of the **aorta** illustrating the appearance of a large elastic artery. H and E. x65.

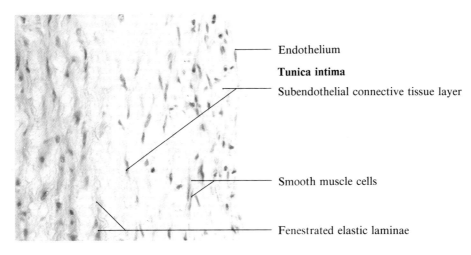

Endothelium

Tunica intima

Subendothelial connective tissue layer

Smooth muscle cells

Fenestrated elastic laminae

Fig. 9-2. Longitudinal section through the wall of the **aorta** showing the tunica intima and innermost part of the tunica media. Note the thick subendothelial connective tissue layer. H and E. x275.

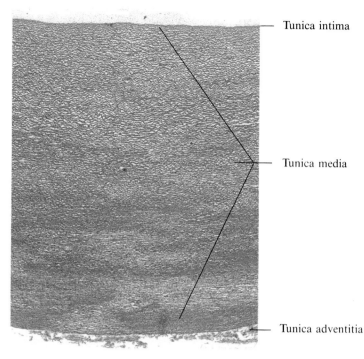

—— Tunica intima

—— Tunica media

—— Tunica adventitia

Fig. 9-3. Part of a cross section through the wall of the **aorta** in which the fenestrated elastic laminae of the tunica media are stained selectively with orcein. x35.

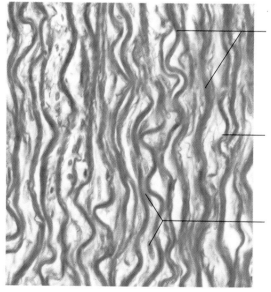

—— Fenestrated elastic laminae

—— Fenestration

—— Smooth muscle cells

Fig. 9-4. Part of the **tunica media of the aorta** showing the densely packed fenestrated elastic laminae. Orcein staining. x440.

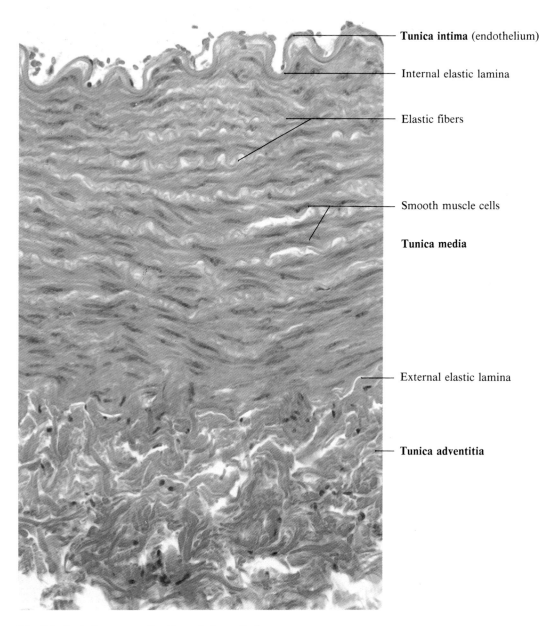

Tunica intima (endothelium)

Internal elastic lamina

Elastic fibers

Smooth muscle cells

Tunica media

External elastic lamina

Tunica adventitia

Fig. 9-5. Part of a cross section through the wall of
a **muscular artery.** H and E. x350.

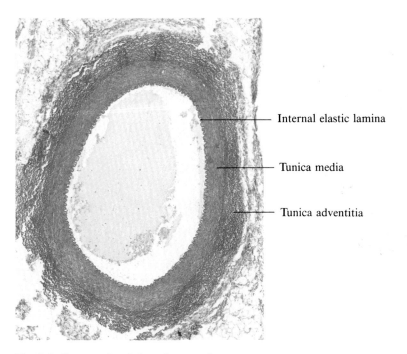

— Internal elastic lamina

— Tunica media

— Tunica adventitia

Fig. 9-6. Cross sectional view of a **muscular artery.**
Orcein staining. x35.

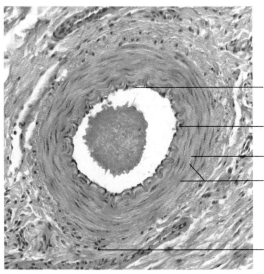

— **Tunica intima** (endothelium)

— Internal elastic lamina

— **Tunica media**

— Smooth muscle cells

— **Tunica adventitia**

Fig. 9-7. Cross sectional view of a small **muscular
artery.** H and E. x165.

External elastic lamina   Internal elastic lamina
Tunica media | Tunica adventitia |

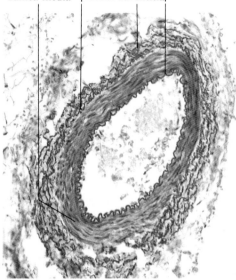

Tunica adventitia   Smooth muscle cells of media
| Endothelium | Internal elastic lamina

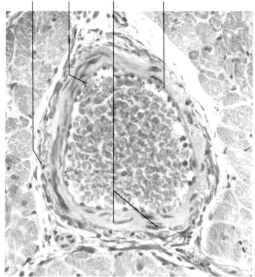

Fig. 9-8. Cross sectional view of a small **muscular artery.** Orcein staining. x165.

Fig. 9-9. Cross sectional view of a very small **muscular artery.** Azan. x275.

Smooth muscle cells of media
            Internal elastic lamina
      Endothelium

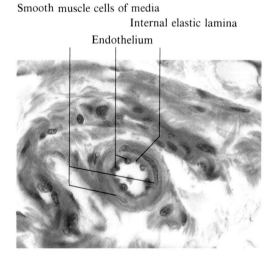

Capillary   Small arterioles   Collecting venule

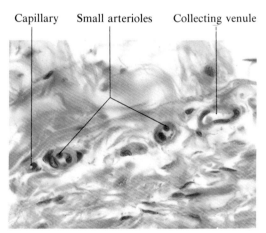

Fig. 9-10. Cross sectional view of an **arteriole,** having two layers of smooth muscle cells in the media. Note that the internal elastic lamina may be seen distinctly in arterial blood vessels even of this small size. H and E. x540.

Fig. 9-11. In this illustration, the histological appearance of the small blood vessels constituting the **microvascular bed** may be compared. H and E. x440.

Cardiac muscle fibers   Capillaries

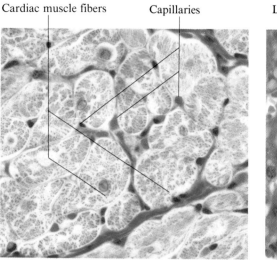

Liver cell cords   Sinusoids

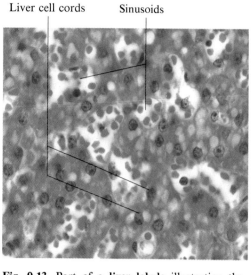

Fig. 9-12. Part of a cross section through the **myo-cardium** in which numerous capillaries are seen between the cardiac muscle fibers. Azan. x540.

Fig. 9-13. Part of a **liver lobule** illustrating the appearance of sinusoids. Note the large size of the sinusoids compared to the capillaries in Fig. 9-12. H and E. x540.

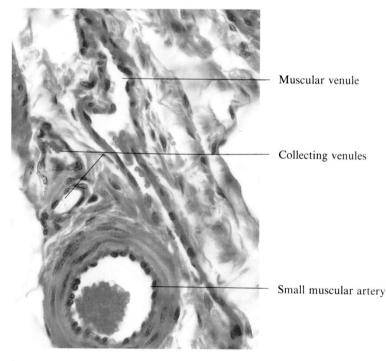

— Muscular venule

— Collecting venules

— Small muscular artery

Fig. 9-14. In this section is shown the characteristic appearance of **venules.** H and E. x440.

Endothelium   Tunica adventitia   Tunica media

Tunica media   Tunica adventitia

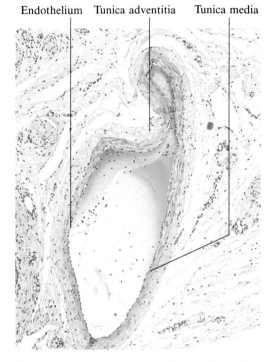

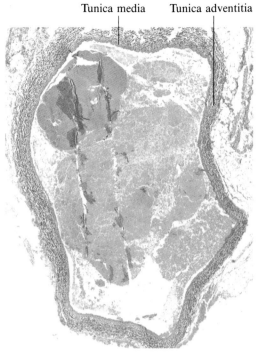

Fig. 9-15. Cross-sectioned **small vein.** Note the partly collapsed appearance. H and E. x65.

Fig. 9-16. Cross sectional view of a **medium-sized vein.** Orcein staining. x25.

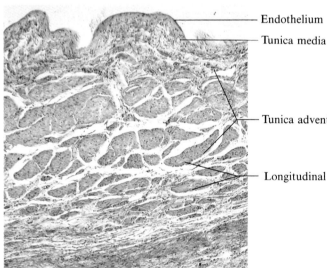

Endothelium

Tunica media

Tunica adventitia

Longitudinal smooth muscle

Fig. 9-17. Part of a transverse section through the wall of a **large vein** (the **inferior caval vein**). Note the very thick tunica adventitia which contains longitudinally oriented bundles of smooth muscle cells. H and E. x65.

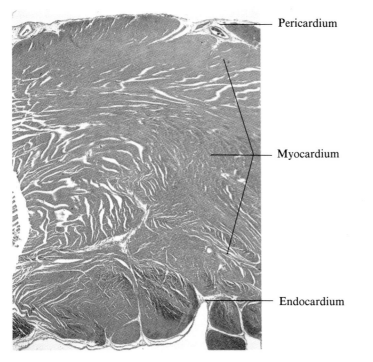

Pericardium

Myocardium

Endocardium

Fig. 9-18. Part of the wall of the **left ventricle of the heart.** H and E. x6.

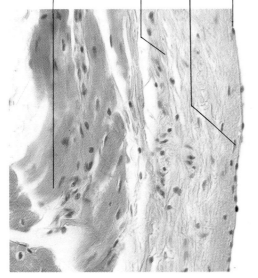

Smooth muscle cell

Myocardium Subendocardial layer Endothelium

Fig. 9-19. Section through the **endocardium** and the innermost part of the myocardium. Note the thick subendocardial layer of connective tissue. H and E. x275.

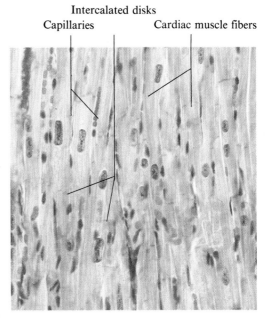

Intercalated disks

Capillaries Cardiac muscle fibers

Fig. 9-20. Longitudinal section through the **myocardium.** Azan. x275.

Myocardium
    Small artery   Fat cells   Nerve

Myocardium   Purkinje fiber   Endothelium

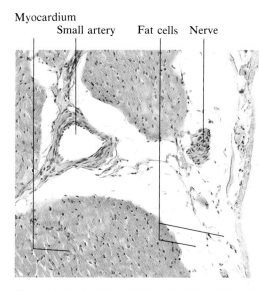

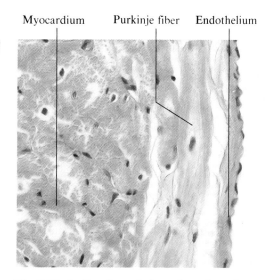

Fig. 9-21. Section through the **epicardium** (visceral layer of the pericardium) and the outermost part of the myocardium. H and E. x110.

Fig. 9-22. Section through the endocardium showing the appearance of a **Purkinje fiber.** H and E. x340.

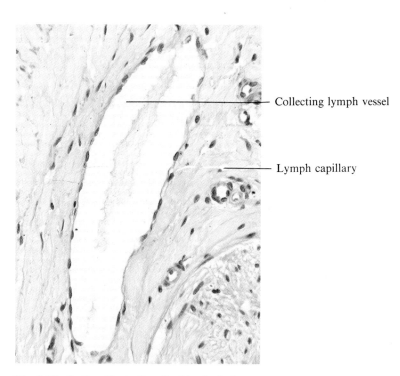

Collecting lymph vessel

Lymph capillary

Fig. 9-23. Section illustrating the histological appearance of small **lymph vessels.** Note the very thin tunica media. H and E. x275.

CHAPTER 10

The Lymphoid Organs

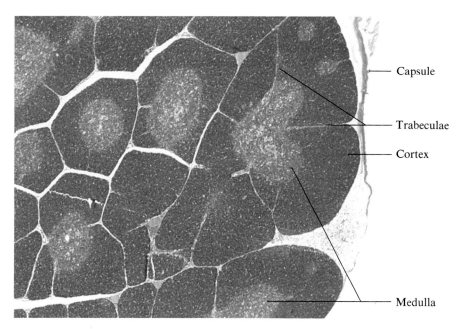

Fig. 10-1. Section through the superficial part of the **thymus** from a child showing no signs of involution. H and E. x25.

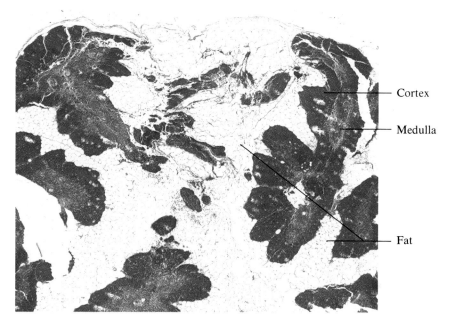

Fig. 10-2. Section through the superficial part of the **thymus** from an adult showing pronounced age involution. Note that a large part of the parenchyme has been replaced by fat. H and E. x20.

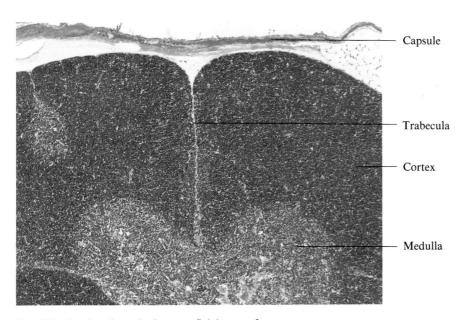

Capsule

Trabecula

Cortex

Medulla

Fig. 10-3. Section through the superficial part of the **thymus** from a child showing the sharp transition between the cortex and medulla. H and E. x65.

Lymphocytes Reticular cells **Cortex** **Medulla**

Thymic corpuscles (of Hassal)

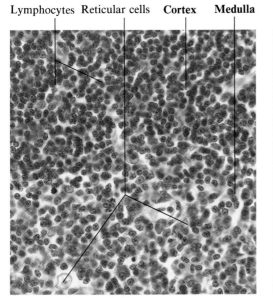

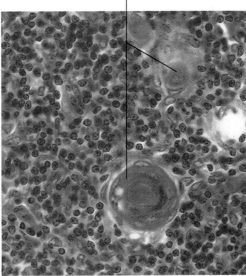

Fig. 10-4. Section showing part of the cortex and medulla of the **thymus.** Note the very large, lightly stained nuclei of the epithelial reticular cells. Note also, the more densely packed lymphocytes in the cortex, causing its darker appearance, as compared to the medulla. H and E. x440.

Fig. 10-5. Part of the **medulla of the thymus** showing two thymic corpuscles (of Hassal). H and E. x440.

Lymphoid nodules in outer cortex   Efferent lymph vessel
Medullary cords   Deep cortex (paracortex)   Hilus

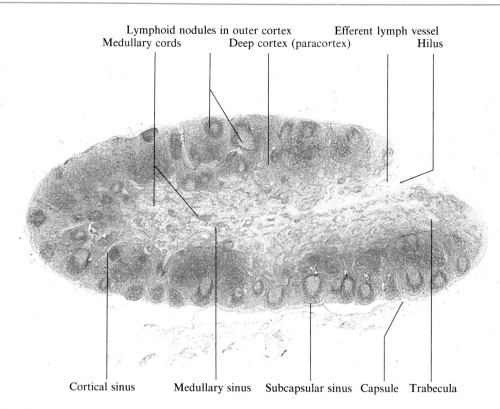

Cortical sinus   Medullary sinus   Subcapsular sinus   Capsule   Trabecula

Fig. 10-6. Low power view of a transected **lymph node.** H and E. x15.

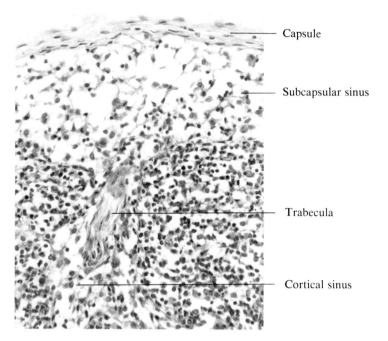

Capsule

Subcapsular sinus

Trabecula

Cortical sinus

Fig. 10-7. Section through the superficial part of a
lymph node. H and E. x275.

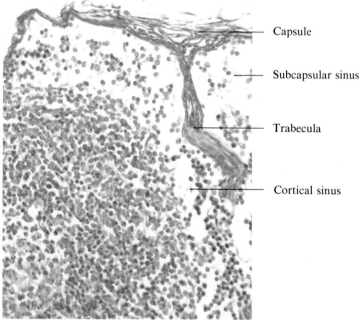

Capsule

Subcapsular sinus

Trabecula

Cortical sinus

Fig. 10-8. Section through the superficial part of a
lymph node. Van Gieson. x275.

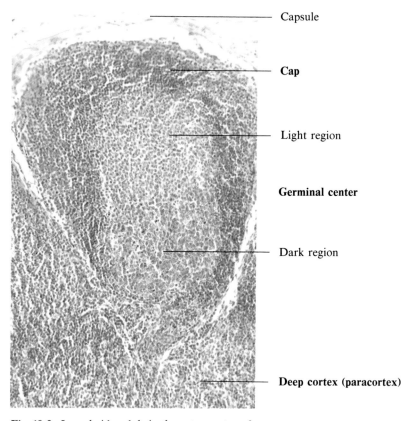

Capsule

Cap

Light region

Germinal center

Dark region

Deep cortex (paracortex)

Fig. 10-9. Lymphoid nodule in the **outer cortex of a lymph node.** H and E. x135.

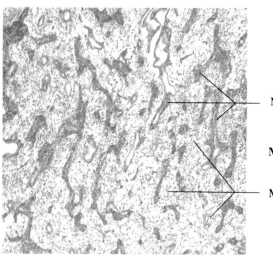

Medullary cords

Medulla

Medullary sinuses

Fig. 10-10. Section through the **medulla of a lymph node.** Van Gieson. x45.

Medullary cords   Medullary sinuses   Reticular fibers   Germinal center

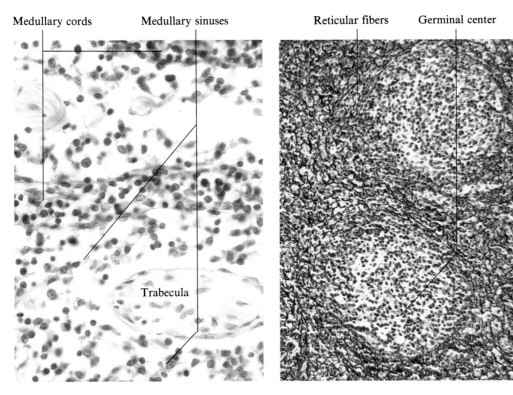

Fig. 10-11. High power view of the **medulla of a lymph node.** H and E. x440.

Fig. 10-12. Section through the **cortex of a lymph node** in which the network of reticular fibers has been demonstrated by means of silver impregnation. Note the absence of fibers in the germinal centers. Bielschowsky. x165.

Lymphocytes
  Macrophages with phagocytosed coal dust   Cuboidal endothelium   **Postcapillary venule**

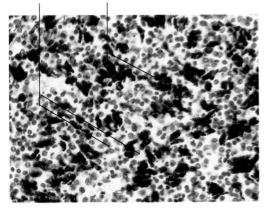
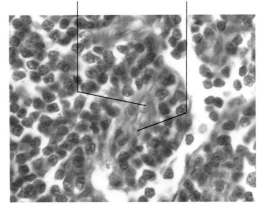

Fig. 10-13. Part of the medulla of a **bronchial lymph node** showing pronounced anthracosis. Thus, the macrophages are loaded with phagocytosed coal dust. H and E. x275.

Fig. 10-14. Postcapillary venule in the **deep cortex (paracortex) of a lymph node.** Note the cuboidal endothelium. H and E. x660.

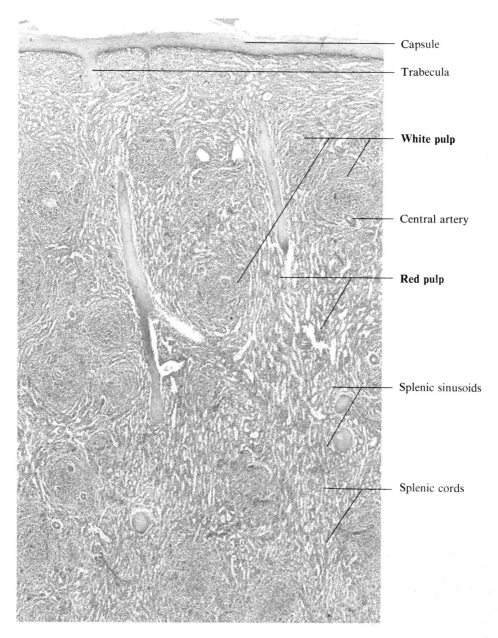

Capsule

Trabecula

White pulp

Central artery

Red pulp

Splenic sinusoids

Splenic cords

Fig. 10-15. Section through the superficial part of the **spleen.** H and E. x30.

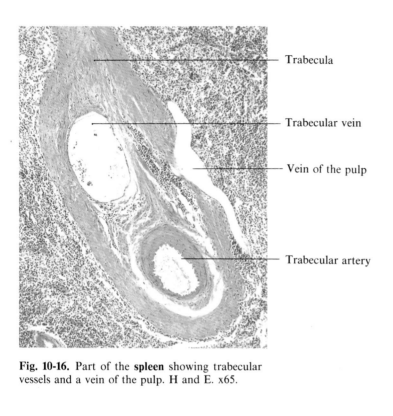

Trabecula

Trabecular vein

Vein of the pulp

Trabecular artery

Fig. 10-16. Part of the **spleen** showing trabecular vessels and a vein of the pulp. H and E. x65.

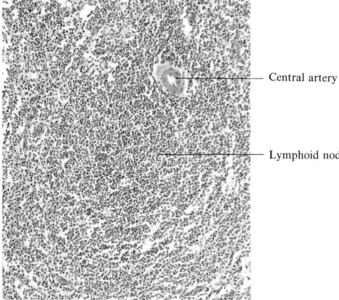

Central artery

Lymphoid nodule (Malpighian body)

Fig. 10-17. Part of the **spleen** showing the appearance of the white pulp. H and E. x110.

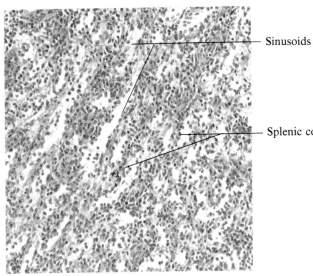

Sinusoids

Splenic cords (of Billroth)

Fig. 10-18. Part of the **spleen** illustrating the appearance of the red pulp. H and E. x165.

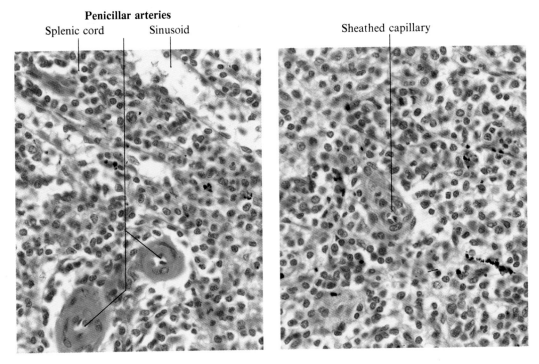

Penicillar arteries

Splenic cord   Sinusoid   Sheathed capillary

Fig. 10-19. High power view of the **red pulp of the spleen.** H and E. x440.

Fig. 10-20. Sheathed capillary in the **red pulp of the spleen.** H and E. x440.

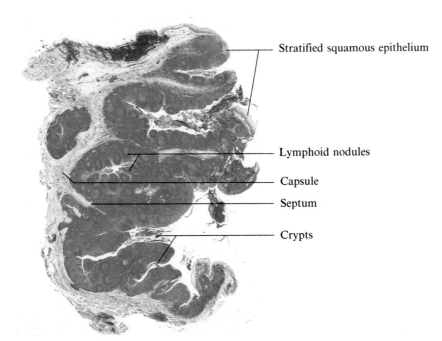

Stratified squamous epithelium

Lymphoid nodules

Capsule

Septum

Crypts

Fig. 10-21. Low power view of a transected **palatine tonsil.** H and E. x5.

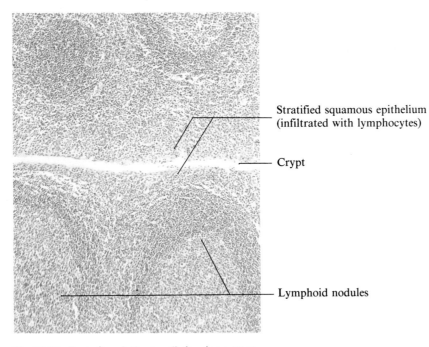

Stratified squamous epithelium
(infiltrated with lymphocytes)

Crypt

Lymphoid nodules

Fig. 10-22. Part of a **palatine tonsil** showing a crypt and its immediate surroundings. H and E. x65.

CHAPTER 11
The Skin

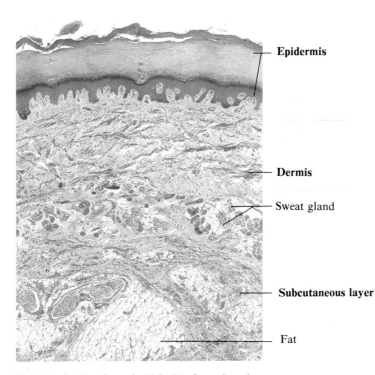

Epidermis

Dermis

Sweat gland

Subcutaneous layer

Fat

Fig. 11-1. Section through **thick skin** from the sole of the foot. Note that the histological term thick skin refers to the very thick epidermis. H and E. x30.

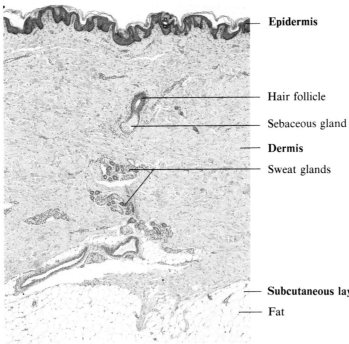

Epidermis

Hair follicle

Sebaceous gland

Dermis

Sweat glands

Subcutaneous layer

Fat

Fig. 11-2. Section through **thin skin** from the abdomen. Note the thin epidermis compared to that in Fig. 11-1. H and E. x30.

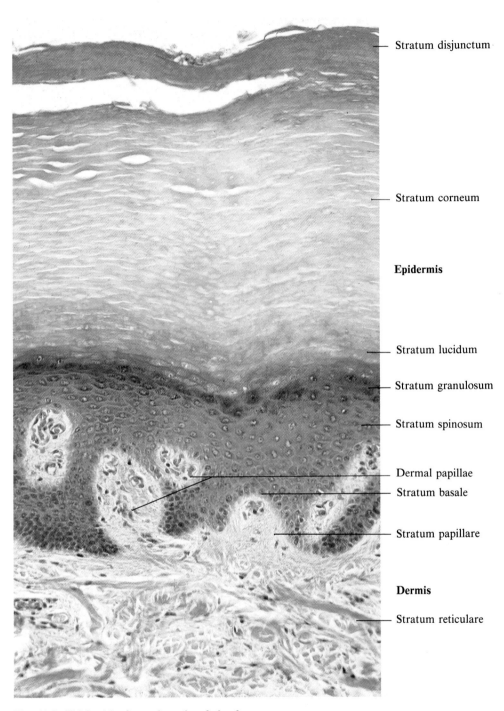

— Stratum disjunctum

— Stratum corneum

Epidermis

— Stratum lucidum

— Stratum granulosum

— Stratum spinosum

— Dermal papillae

— Stratum basale

— Stratum papillare

Dermis

— Stratum reticulare

Fig. 11-3. Thick skin from the sole of the foot, illustrating the layers of the epidermis. Moreover, the papillary and reticular layers of the dermis are seen. H and E. x220.

Intercellular bridges   Keratohyalin granules

Stratum granulosum
                Melanin granules   Clear cell

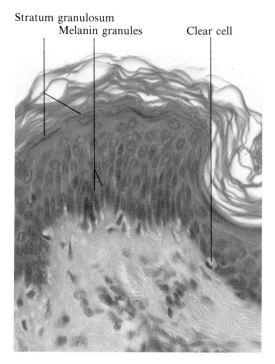

Fig. 11-4. High power view of part of the **epidermis of thick skin.** H and E. x660.

Fig. 11-5. High power view of the **epidermis of thin skin.** Note the very thin stratum granulosum and corneum and the absence of the stratum lucidum. Note too, the presence of melanin granules in the supranuclear cytoplasm of many of the keratinocytes. Moreover, a clear cell (melanocyte) is seen. H and E. x440.

Processes   Melanocyte

Melanocytes

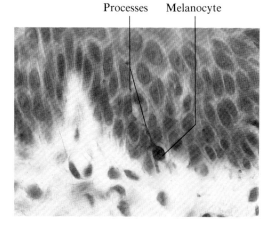

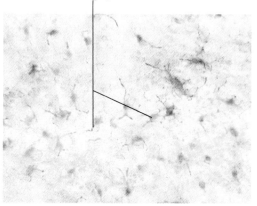

Fig. 11-6. High power view of the heavily pigmented **epidermis** of a monkey, showing a melanocyte containing melanin. Note the clear space around the cell body of the melanocyte and the long dendritic processes. H and E. x660.

Fig. 11-7. Preparation of the **epidermis** (from a biopsy of the skin of the face) which has been stripped from the dermis and exposed to the DOPA reaction for the histochemical demonstration of melanocytes. Note the branching processes of the melanocytes, forming an almost continuous network in the basal part of the epidermis. x275.

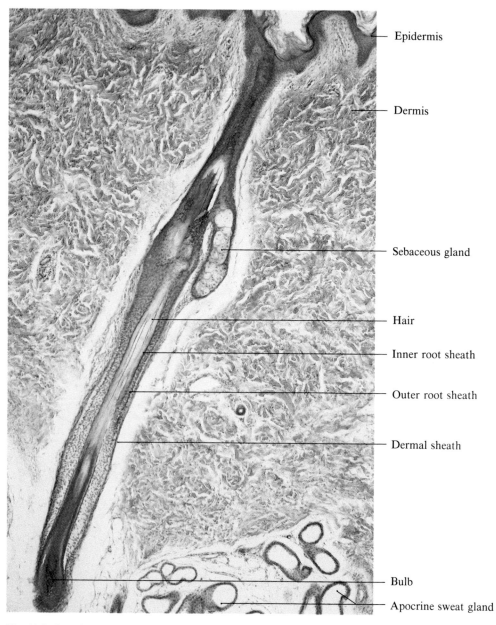

Epidermis

Dermis

Sebaceous gland

Hair

Inner root sheath

Outer root sheath

Dermal sheath

Bulb

Apocrine sweat gland

Fig. 11-8. Longitudinal section through the **root of a hair and associated hair follicle.** H and E. x65.

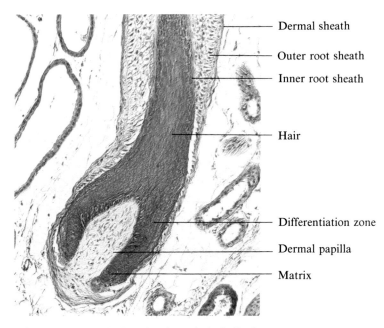

Dermal sheath

Outer root sheath

Inner root sheath

Hair

Differentiation zone

Dermal papilla

Matrix

Fig. 11-9. Longitudinal section through the **bulb of a hair.** H and E. x110.

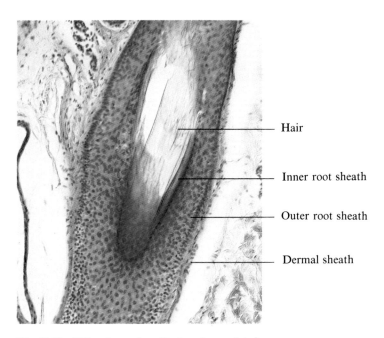

Hair

Inner root sheath

Outer root sheath

Dermal sheath

Fig. 11-10. Obliquely-sectioned **hair and associated hair follicle.** H and E. x110.

Hyponychium   Nail   Nail bed   Eponychium

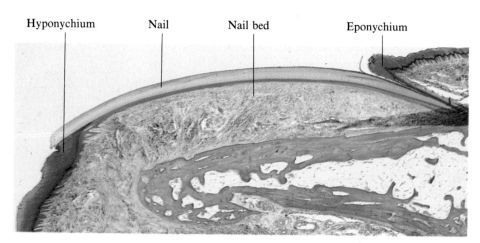

Fig. 11-11. Longitudinal section through a **nail and nail bed.** H and E. x7.

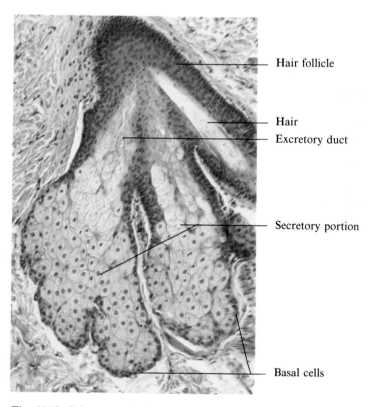

Hair follicle

Hair
Excretory duct

Secretory portion

Basal cells

Fig. 11-12. Sebaceous gland and associated hair follicle. H and E. x135.

Apocrine sweat gland
Excretory duct   Secretory portion   Secretory cells   Myoepithelial cells

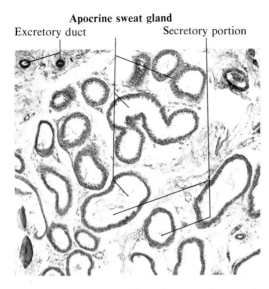

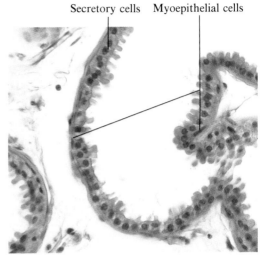

Fig. 11-13. Low power view of an **apocrine sweat gland of the axilla.** H and E. x55.

Fig. 11-14. Part of the secretory portion of an **apocrine sweat gland.** Note the characteristic protrusions of the apical cytoplasm of the secretory cells. These protrusions are (to some extent) pinched off by the apocrine secretory mechanism of this type of gland. H and E. x275.

Secretory portion
Myoepithelial cells   Excretory duct

Excretory duct (epidermal course)
            Excretory duct (dermal part)

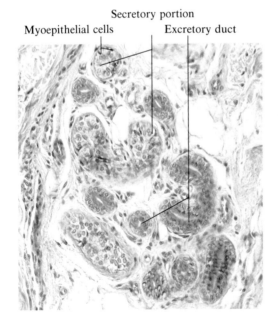

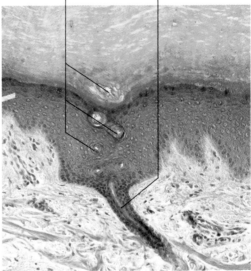

Fig. 11-15. Secretory portion and initial portion of the excretory duct of an **eccrine sweat gland.** H and E. x165.

Fig. 11-16. Excretory duct of an eccrine sweat gland where it enters the epidermis corresponding to a deep epidermal ridge. The wall of the corkscrew-shaped duct in the epidermis is formed by the epidermal cells, since the excretory duct loses its own wall at the transition to the epidermis. H and E. x135.

CHAPTER 12

The Digestive System

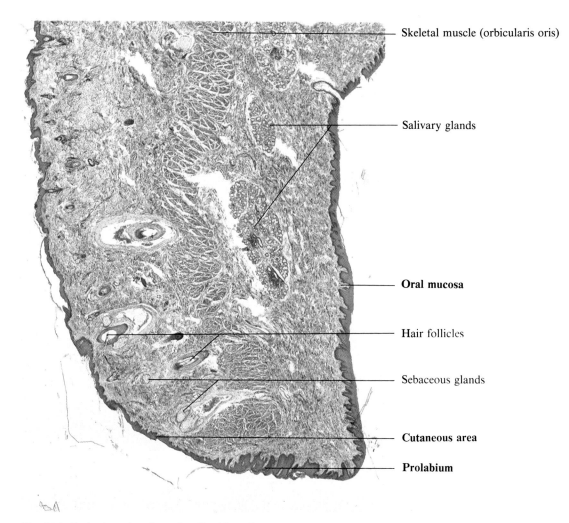

Skeletal muscle (orbicularis oris)

Salivary glands

Oral mucosa

Hair follicles

Sebaceous glands

Cutaneous area

Prolabium

Fig. 12-1. Sagittal section through a **lip.** Note the very high connective tissue papillae in the prolabium (the red part of the lip). H and E. x15.

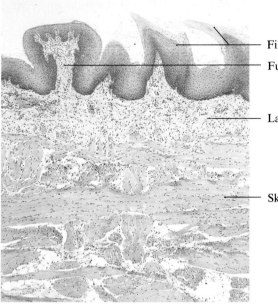

Filiform papillae

Fungiform papilla

Lamina propria

Skeletal muscle

Fig. 12-2. Section through the dorsal surface of the oral part of the **tongue** showing a fungiform and two filiform papillae. H and E. x45.

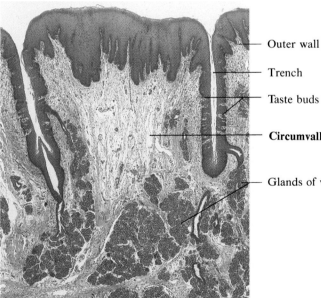

Outer wall

Trench

Taste buds

Circumvallate papilla

Glands of von Ebner

Fig. 12-3. Section through the dorsal surface of the oral part of the **tongue** showing a circumvallate papilla. H and E. x30.

Foliate papilla   Taste buds

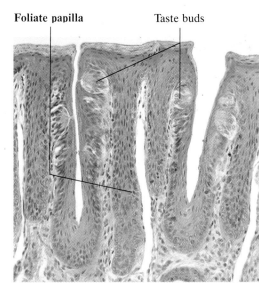

Taste bud   Taste pore

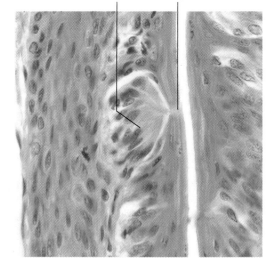

Fig. 12-4. Foliate papilla from the **tongue** of a rabbit. H and E. x165.

Fig. 12-5. High power view of a taste bud from the **tongue.** H and E. x540.

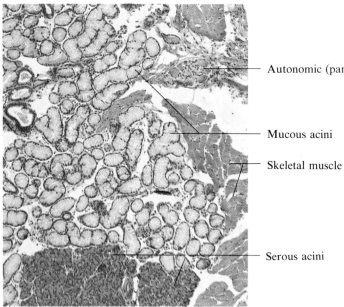

— Autonomic (parasympathetic) ganglion

— Mucous acini

— Skeletal muscle

— Serous acini

Fig. 12-6. Part of the **anterior lingual gland** showing mucous and serous secretory portions. H and E. x65.

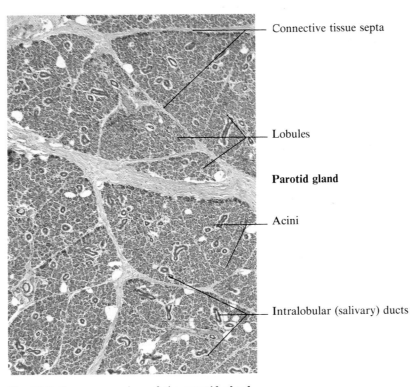

Connective tissue septa

Lobules

Parotid gland

Acini

Intralobular (salivary) ducts

Fig. 12-7. Low power view of the **parotid gland** showing the characteristic lobulation. H and E. x45.

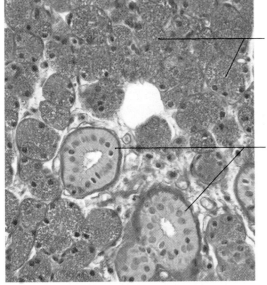

Serous acini

Parotid gland

Salivary (striated) ducts

Fig. 12-8. Part of the **parotid gland,** seen at higher power, showing serous acini and salivary ducts. Van Gieson. x275.

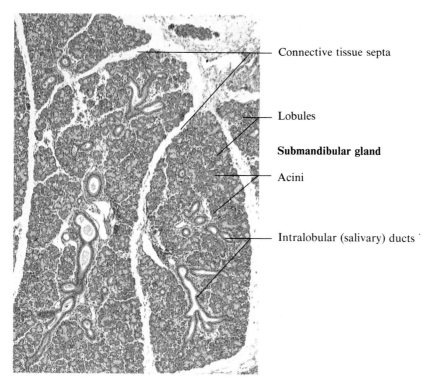

Connective tissue septa

Lobules

Submandibular gland

Acini

Intralobular (salivary) ducts

Fig. 12-9. Low power view of the **submandibular gland** showing the unusually well developed long salivary ducts. H and E. x45.

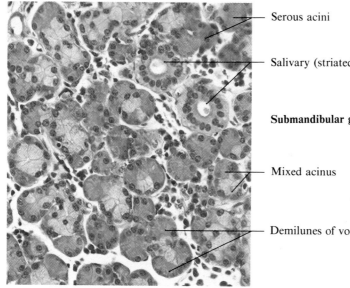

Serous acini

Salivary (striated) ducts

Submandibular gland

Mixed acinus

Demilunes of von Ebner

Fig. 12-10. Part of the **submandibular gland,** seen at higher power, showing the predominantly serous character of this mixed seromucous gland. H and E. x275.

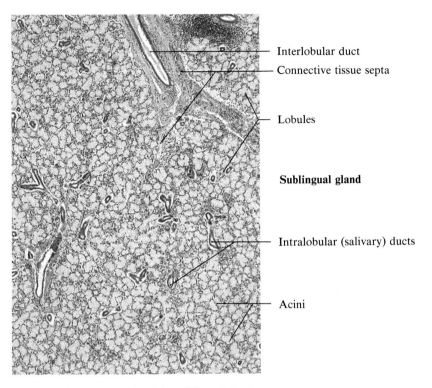

Interlobular duct

Connective tissue septa

Lobules

Sublingual gland

Intralobular (salivary) ducts

Acini

Fig. 12-11. Low power view of the **sublingual gland.**
H and E. x45.

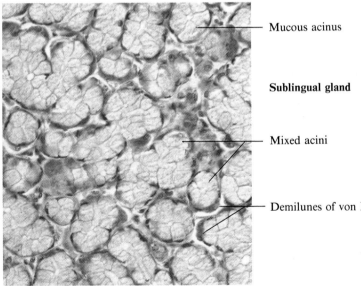

Mucous acinus

Sublingual gland

Mixed acini

Demilunes of von Ebner

Fig. 12-12. Part of the **sublingual gland,** seen at
higher power, showing the predominantly mucous
character of this mixed mucoserous gland. H and
E. x275.

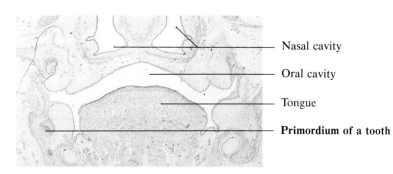

Nasal cavity

Oral cavity

Tongue

Primordium of a tooth

Fig. 12-13. Part of a frontal section through the **head of a fetus** showing the primordium of a tooth. H and E. x7.

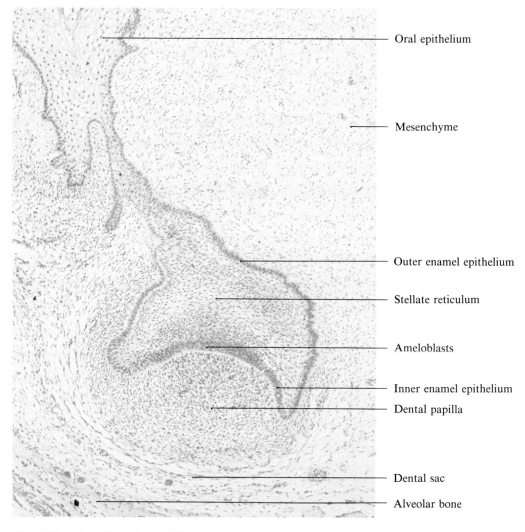

Oral epithelium

Mesenchyme

Outer enamel epithelium

Stellate reticulum

Ameloblasts

Inner enamel epithelium
Dental papilla

Dental sac
Alveolar bone

Fig. 12-14. Primordium of a tooth in the cap stage of development. H and E. x100.

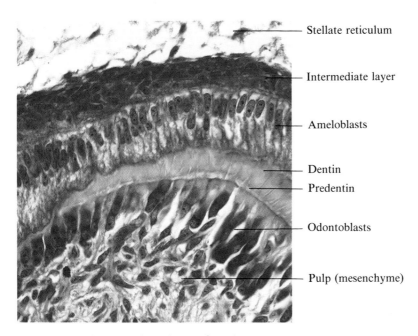

Stellate reticulum

Intermediate layer

Ameloblasts

Dentin
Predentin

Odontoblasts

Pulp (mesenchyme)

Fig. 12-15. High power view of part of a **primordium of a tooth** in the bell stage of development, shortly after the commencement of the formation of dentin. Azan. x540.

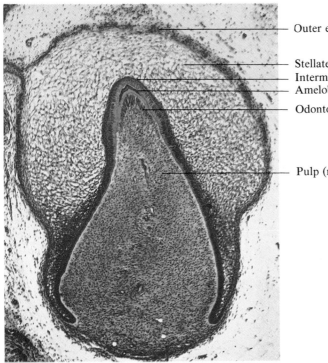

Outer enamel epithelium

Stellate reticulum
Intermediate layer
Ameloblasts

Odontoblasts

Pulp (mesenchyme)

Fig. 12-16. Primordium of a tooth in the bell stage of development. Toluidine blue. x40.

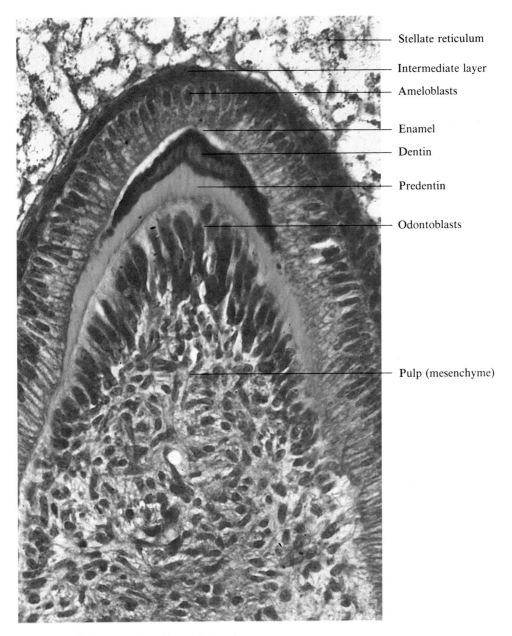

Stellate reticulum

Intermediate layer

Ameloblasts

Enamel

Dentin

Predentin

Odontoblasts

Pulp (mesenchyme)

Fig. 12-17. High power view of part of the **primordium of a tooth** in the bell stage of development, shortly after the commencement of the formation of enamel. Toluidine blue. x415.

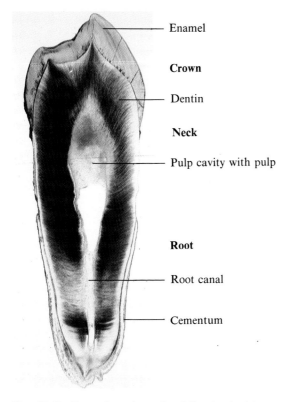

Enamel

Crown

Dentin

Neck

Pulp cavity with pulp

Root

Root canal

Cementum

Fig. 12-18. Ground section of a fully developed **tooth.** x5.

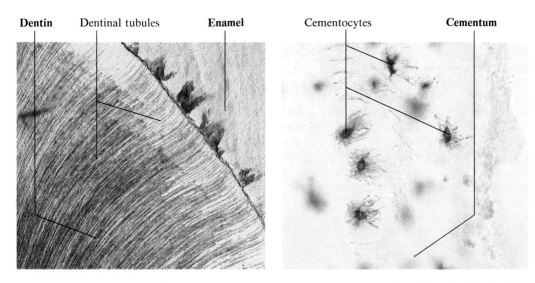

Dentin   Dentinal tubules   **Enamel**

Fig. 12-19. Part of a ground section of a **tooth** showing the dentinoenamel junction. x45.

Cementocytes   **Cementum**

Fig. 12-20. Ground section of a **tooth,** showing the cellular cementum of the apical half of the root. x275.

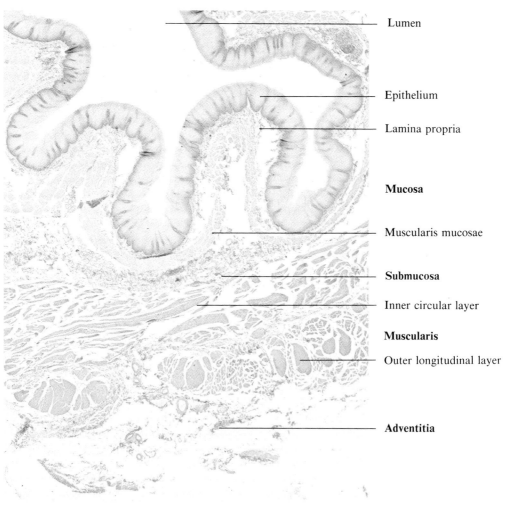

Lumen

Epithelium

Lamina propria

Mucosa

Muscularis mucosae

Submucosa

Inner circular layer

Muscularis

Outer longitudinal layer

Adventitia

Fig. 12-21. Cross sectional view of the wall of the **esophagus.** H and E. x15.

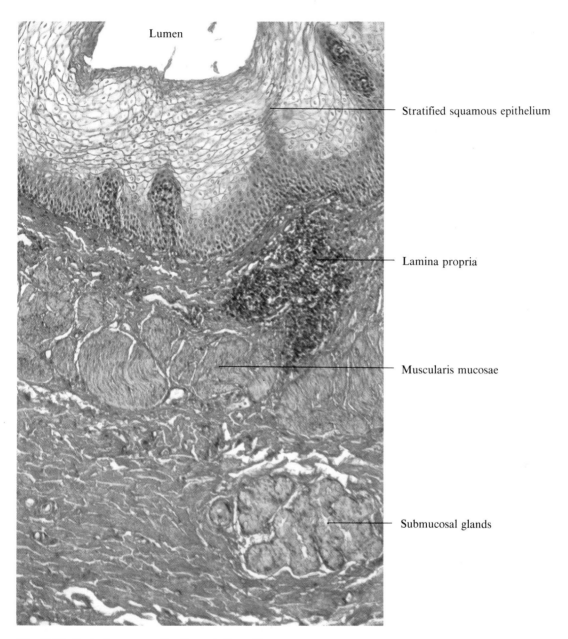

Lumen

Stratified squamous epithelium

Lamina propria

Muscularis mucosae

Submucosal glands

Fig. 12-22. Part of a cross section through the wall of the **esophagus** showing the mucosa and submucosa. Van Gieson. x135.

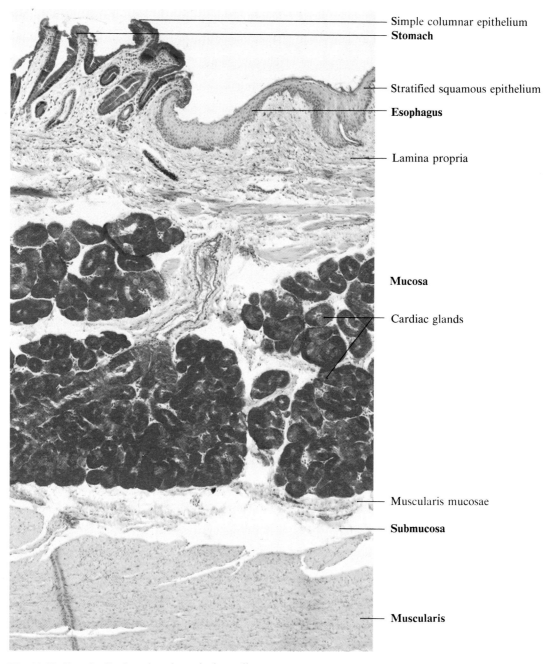

Simple columnar epithelium
Stomach

Stratified squamous epithelium

Esophagus

Lamina propria

Mucosa

Cardiac glands

Muscularis mucosae

Submucosa

Muscularis

Fig. 12-23. Longitudinal section through the wall of the **esophagus** at the transition to the **stomach**. Note the abrupt change of the stratified squamous epithelium of the esophagus into the simple columnar epithelium of the stomach. The cardiac glands and the surface epithelium of the stomach are stained red by using the PAS reaction in this section. PAS + Van Gieson. x90.

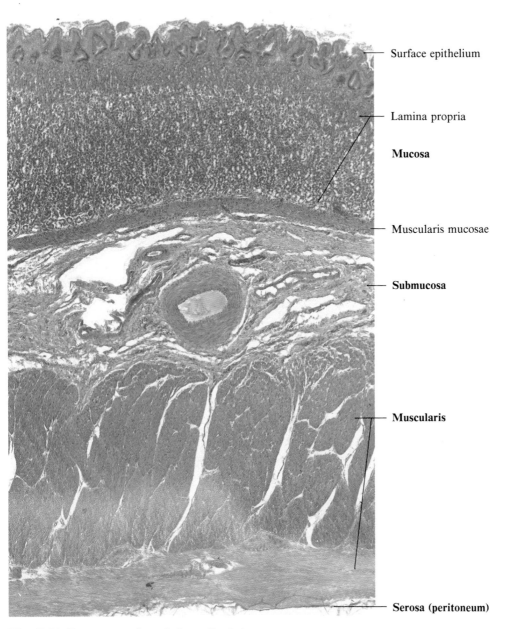

Surface epithelium

Lamina propria

Mucosa

Muscularis mucosae

Submucosa

Muscularis

Serosa (peritoneum)

Fig. 12-24. Low power view of the wall of the **stomach.** H and E. x45.

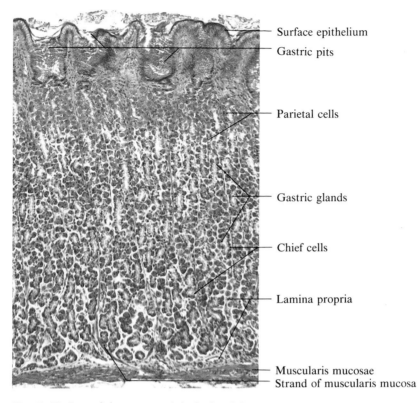

— Surface epithelium
— Gastric pits

— Parietal cells

— Gastric glands

— Chief cells

— Lamina propria

— Muscularis mucosae
— Strand of muscularis mucosa

Fig. 12-25. Part of the **mucosa of the body of the stomach.** H and E. x130.

Surface epithelium

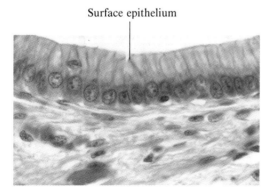

Fig. 12-26. High power view of the **surface epithelium of the stomach.** H and E. x540.

Surface epithelium

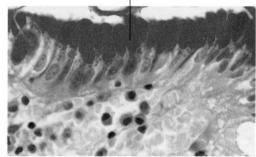

Fig. 12-27. High power view of the **surface epithelium of the stomach,** stained using the PAS reaction. Note that all the cells of the surface epithelium are PAS-positive. They are mucus-secreting and together form a secretory epithelial sheath. PAS + H and E. x540.

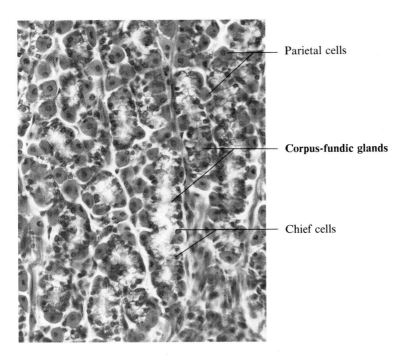

Parietal cells

Corpus-fundic glands

Chief cells

Fig. 12-28. Part of the **mucosa of the body of the stomach** showing the appearance of the corpus-fundic glands when seen at higher power. H and E. x240.

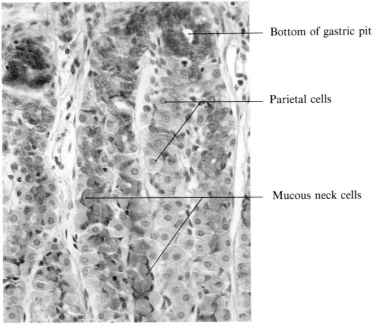

Bottom of gastric pit

Parietal cells

Mucous neck cells

Fig. 12-29. Part of the **mucosa of the body of the stomach,** showing mucus neck cells in the necks of the corpus-fundic glands. The mucus neck cells are stained red by the PAS reaction. PAS + van Gieson. x275.

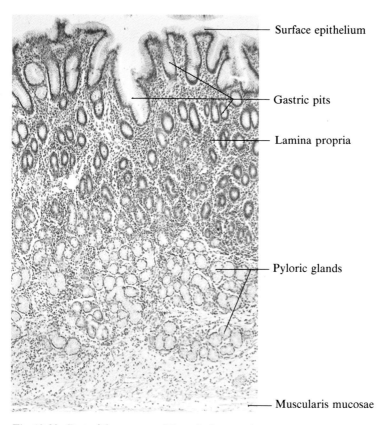

Surface epithelium

Gastric pits

Lamina propria

Pyloric glands

Muscularis mucosae

Fig. 12-30. Part of the **mucosa of the pyloric part of the stomach.** Note the numerous cross sectional profiles of the pyloric glands due to their pronounced coiling. H and E. x75.

Lamina propria Pyloric glands Gastric pit

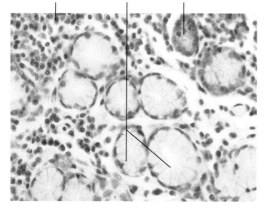

Fig. 12-31. High power view of **pyloric glands** showing their mucous character. Note the different appearance of the bottom of the gastric pit seen in the upper right corner. H and E. x305.

Gastrin-producing (G) cells   Pyloric glands

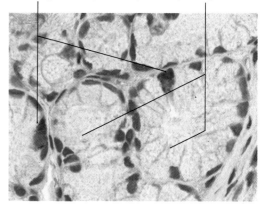

Fig. 12-32. High power view of **pyloric glands** in which the gastrin-producing (G) cells have been demonstrated immunohistochemically. The section was embedded in Epon and counterstained with methylene blue. x550.

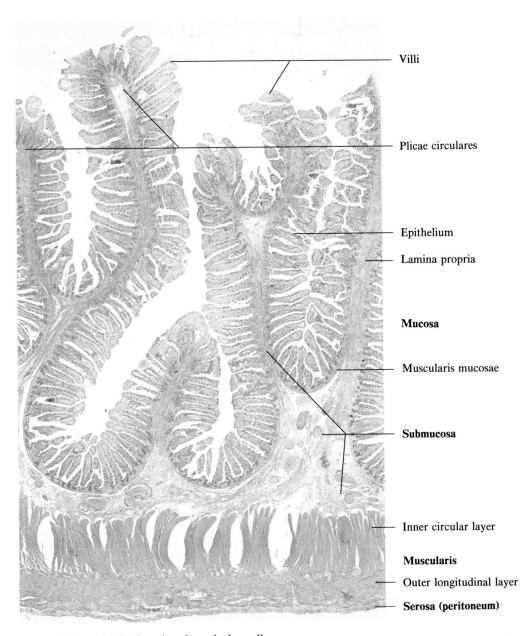

Villi

Plicae circulares

Epithelium

Lamina propria

Mucosa

Muscularis mucosae

Submucosa

Inner circular layer

Muscularis

Outer longitudinal layer

Serosa (peritoneum)

Fig. 12-33. Longitudinal section through the wall of the **jejunal part of the small intestine.** Note the branched plicae circulares of Kerkring which consist of both the mucosa and submucosa and are permanent structures. Van Gieson. x15.

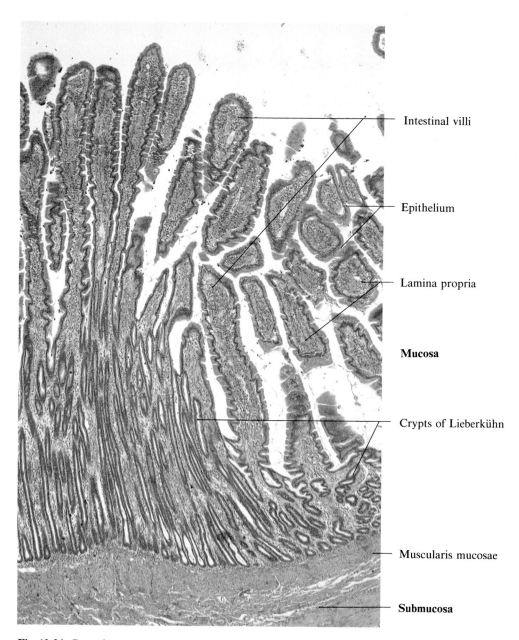

Intestinal villi

Epithelium

Lamina propria

Mucosa

Crypts of Lieberkühn

Muscularis mucosae

Submucosa

Fig. 12-34. Part of a transverse section through the **mucosa of the small intestine.** Note the cross sectioned villi which are seen as epithelium-covered islands of connective tissue. H and E. x65.

Core of villus (lamina propria)
Brush border   Goblet cells

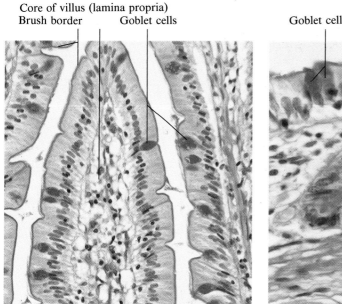

Goblet cells   Paneth cells

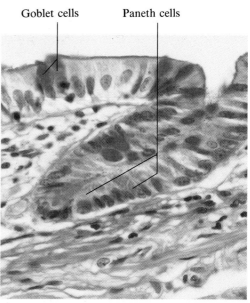

Fig. 12-35. Part of an **intestinal villus** seen at higher power. The goblet cells and the brush border of the absorptive cells are stained red using the PAS reaction. Note the very cellular connective tissue of the lamina propria. PAS + van Gieson. x275.

Fig. 12-36. Small crypt of Lieberkühn of the **small intestinal mucosa.** A number of Paneth cells are seen in the bottom of the crypt. PAS + van Gieson. x540.

Paneth cells   Goblet cells   Endocrine cell

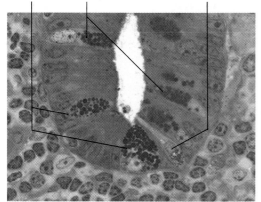

Somatostatin-producing (D) cell
              Intestinal epithelium

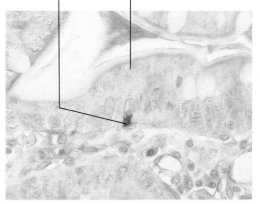

Fig. 12-37. High power view of the bottom of a crypt of Lieberkühn of the **small intestinal mucosa.** In addition to goblet cells, two Paneth cells and an "open type" endocrine cell are seen. Note the fine character of the granules of the endocrine cell and their position in the infranuclear cytoplasm. Epon-embedded section, stained with methylene blue. x660.

Fig. 12-38. High power view of a somatostatin-producing (D) cell of the **mucosa of the small intestine,** demonstrated immunohistochemically. x660.

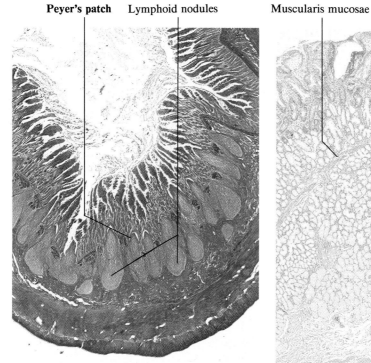

Peyer's patch Lymphoid nodules

Glands of Brunner
Muscularis mucosae   Submucosa

Fig. 12-39. Peyer's patch in the lamina propria of the **mucosa of the ileum.** Azan. x15.

Fig. 12-40. Transverse section through the wall of the **duodenum** showing the glands of Brunner in the submucosa (and the mucosa). H and E. x25.

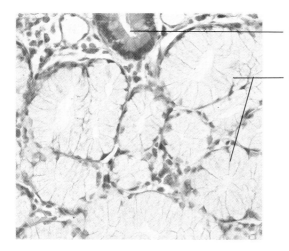

———————— Crypt of Lieberkühn

———— Glands of Brunner

Fig. 12-41. Part of the secretory portion of the **duodenal glands of Brunner.** Note the characteristic mucous appearance of the secretory units. H and E. x275.

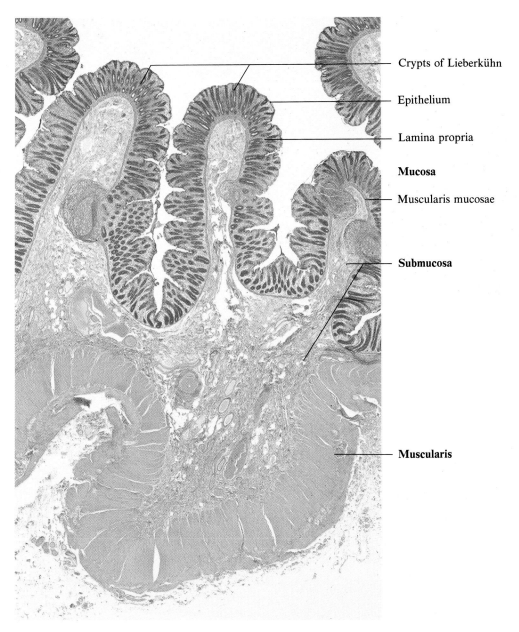

Crypts of Lieberkühn

Epithelium

Lamina propria

Mucosa

Muscularis mucosae

Submucosa

Muscularis

Fig. 12-42. Transverse section through the wall of the **colon.** PAS + van Gieson. x18.

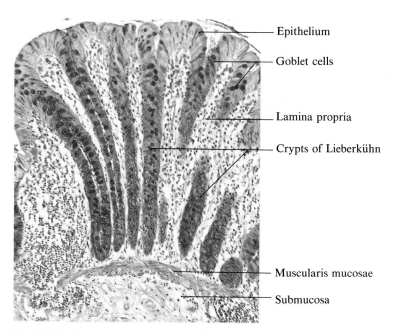

Epithelium

Goblet cells

Lamina propria

Crypts of Lieberkühn

Muscularis mucosae

Submucosa

Fig. 12-43. Transverse section through the wall of the **colon** showing the mucosa and part of the submucosa. Note the straight crypts of Lieberkühn and the abundance of goblet cells (stained red with the PAS reaction). PAS + van Gieson. x110.

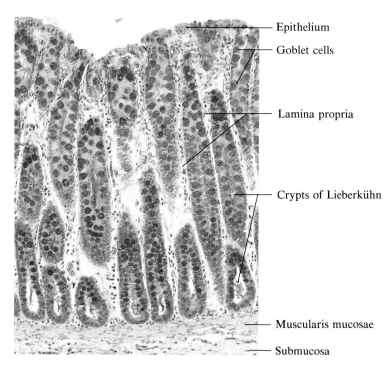

Epithelium

Goblet cells

Lamina propria

Crypts of Lieberkühn

Muscularis mucosae

Submucosa

Fig. 12-44. Transverse section through the wall of the **colon** showing the mucosa and part of the submucosa. The goblet cells are stained red with mucicarmine. Mucicarmine + H and E. x140.

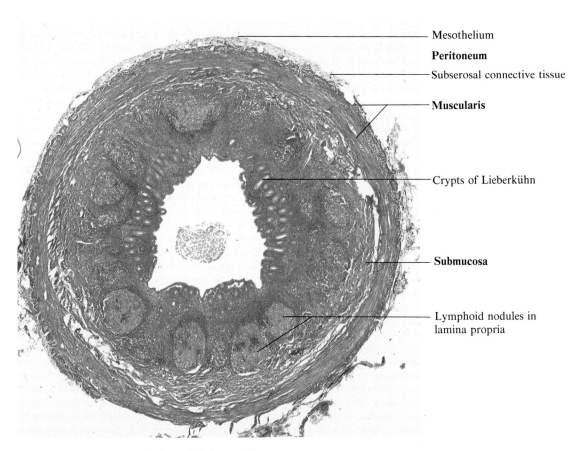

Mesothelium

Peritoneum

Subserosal connective tissue

Muscularis

Crypts of Lieberkühn

Submucosa

Lymphoid nodules in lamina propria

Fig. 12-45. Cross sectional view of the **appendix vermiformis.** Note the irregularly shaped lumen, the paucity of crypts of Lieberkühn and, in particular, the large amount of lymphoid tissue in the lamina propria. H and E. x20.

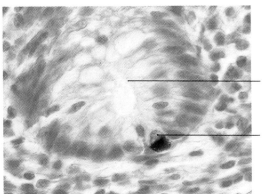

Crypt of Lieberkühn

Argentaffin cell

Fig. 12-46. Argentaffin cell in the bottom of a crypt of Lieberkühn of the **appendix.** The section has been incubated in a basic solution of silver nitrate. This is reduced to metallic silver by serotonin (5-hydroxytryptamine) which occurs in the granules in the basal part of the cell. Therefore, the granules appear darkly stained (the section is counterstained with neutral red). x660.

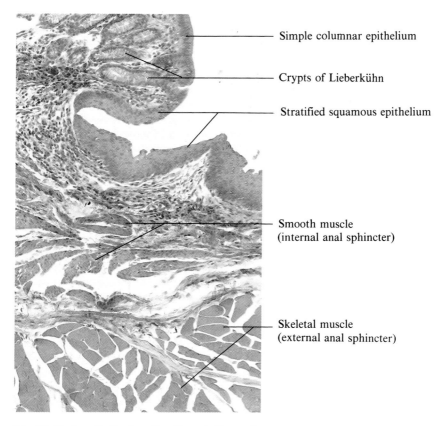

Simple columnar epithelium

Crypts of Lieberkühn

Stratified squamous epithelium

Smooth muscle
(internal anal sphincter)

Skeletal muscle
(external anal sphincter)

Fig. 12-47. Longitudinal section through the **anal canal** at the level of the pectinate line. Note the abrupt transition from simple columnar epithelium to stratified squamous. H and E. x135.

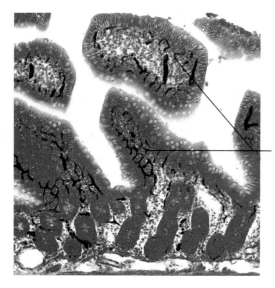

Capillary plexuses

Fig. 12-48. Section of the **small intestinal mucosa** showing the capillary plexuses in the villi. Prior to the preparation of the section, Indian ink was injected into the intestinal arteries of the living, anaesthetized experimental animal. Note that the Indian ink-filled blood capillaries in the villi are situated immediately beneath the epithelium. The section is counterstained with neutral red. x110.

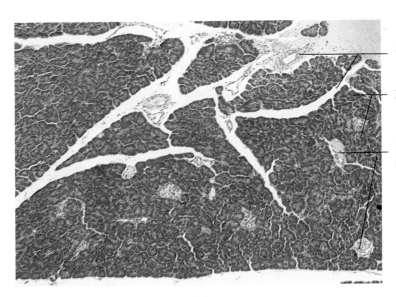

Connective tissue septa

Exocrine tissue (acini)

Endocrine tissue
(Islets of Langerhans)

Fig. 12-49. Low power view of part of the **pancreas** showing the distribution of exocrine and endocrine tissue. H and E. x65.

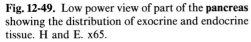

Centroacinar cells
Islet of Langerhans
Acini

Interlobular excretory duct

Acini
Islets of Langerhans

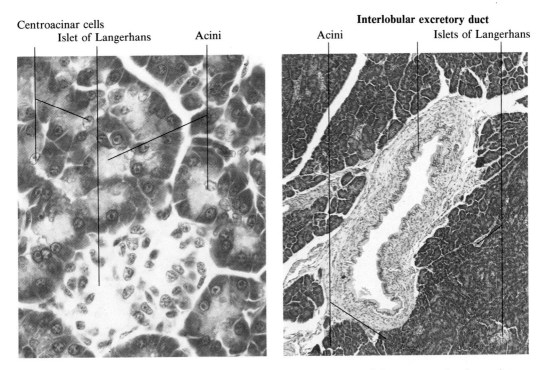

Fig. 12-50. High power view of part of the **pancreas** showing exocrine acini and an islet of Langerhans. Note the rather uniform appearance of the islet cells. H and E. x565.

Fig. 12-51. Part of the **pancreas** showing an inter-lobular excretory duct. H and E. x65.

Glucagon-secreting (A) cells   Islet of Langerhans

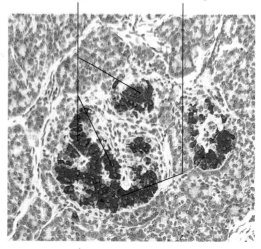

Insulin-secreting (B) cells   Islet of Langerhans

Fig. 12-52. This and the following three pictures show consecutive serial sections of the same islet of Langerhans of a human **pancreas.** In the section in this picture, the distribution of the glucagon-secreting (A) cells has been demonstrated immunohistochemically. Note the occurrence of the A cells throughout the islet as it is characteristic of the human pancreas. Epon-embedded section, counterstained with methylene blue. x135.

Fig. 12-53. Part of a human **pancreas** showing the distribution of insulin-secreting (B) cells in an islet of Langerhans. The B cells were stained immunohistochemically. Epon-embedded section, counterstained with methylene blue. x135.

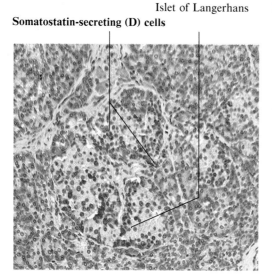

Islet of Langerhans
Somatostatin-secreting (D) cells

Pancreatic polypeptide-secreting (PP) cells
Islet of Langerhans

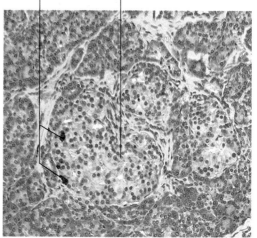

Fig. 12-54. Part of a human **pancreas** showing the distribution of somatostatin-secreting (D) cells in an islet of Langerhans. The D cells were stained immunohistochemically. Epon-embedded section, counterstained with methylene blue. x135.

Fig. 12-55. Part of a human **pancreas** showing the distribution of pancreatic polypeptide-secreting (PP) cells in an islet of Langerhans. The PP cells were stained immunohistochemically. Epon-embedded section, counterstained with methylene blue. x135.

124

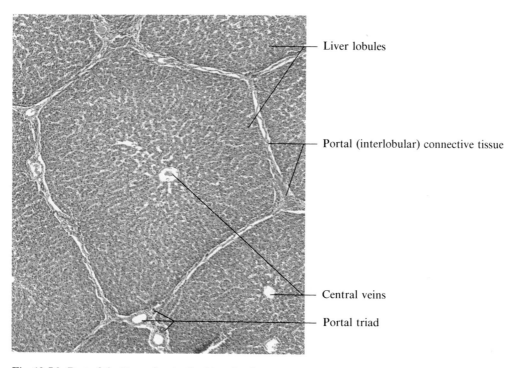

— Liver lobules

— Portal (interlobular) connective tissue

— Central veins

— Portal triad

Fig. 12-56. Part of the **liver** of a pig. In this animal species, the delimitation of the liver lobules is especially distinct due to the abundant interlobular connective tissue. H and E. x55.

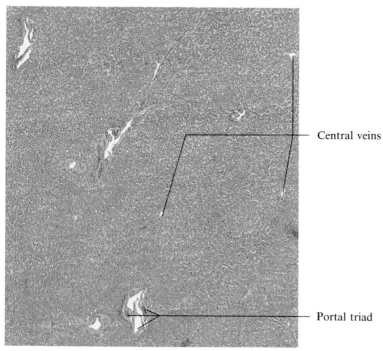

— Central veins

— Portal triad

Fig. 12-57. Part of the **liver** of an ox. The interlobular connective tissue is present in very scant amounts in this animal species (as in Man and most mammalian species) and accordingly the liver parenchyme forms a continuous mass without distinct delimitation of the lobules (cp. Fig. 12-56). H and E. x45.

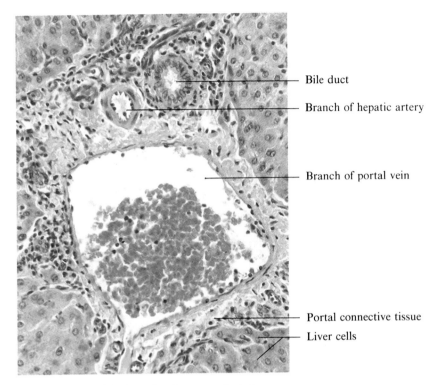

Bile duct

Branch of hepatic artery

Branch of portal vein

Portal connective tissue

Liver cells

Fig. 12-58. Part of the **liver** showing a portal triad.
H and E. x275.

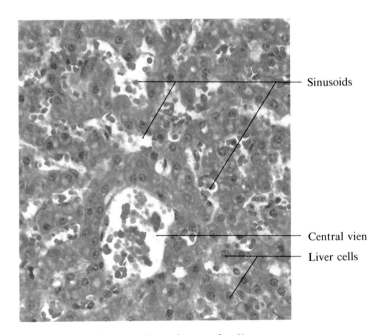

Sinusoids

Central vien

Liver cells

Fig. 12-59. High power view of part of a **liver lobule** showing cords of liver cells, sinusoids and a central vein. H and E. x340.

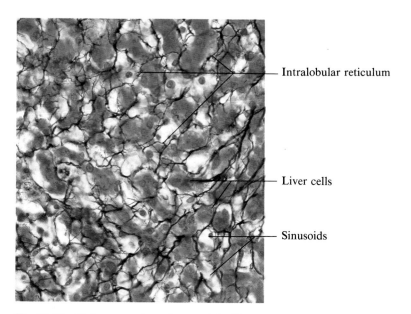

Intralobular reticulum

Liver cells

Sinusoids

Fig. 12-60. High power view of part of the **liver.** The intralobular network of reticular fibers has been demonstrated by silver impregnation and the section is counterstained with eosin. Bielschowsky staining. x275.

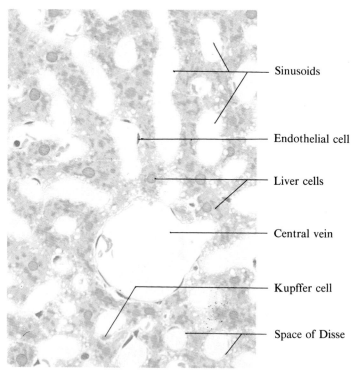

Sinusoids

Endothelial cell

Liver cells

Central vein

Kupffer cell

Space of Disse

Fig. 12-61. High power view of the central part of a **liver lobule.** Metachrylate-embedded section, stained with hematoxylin and eosin. x440.

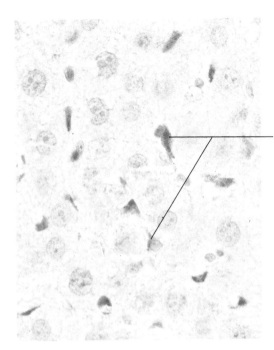

Kupffer cells
containing phagocytosed
lithium carmine

Fig. 12-62. Section of **liver** in which the Kupffer cells have been stained vitally with lithium carmine. This was injected into the portal vein of the living animal prior to the preparation of the section, and has been taken up by phagocytosis of the Kupffer cells which appear red (the section is counter-stained with hematoxylin). x660.

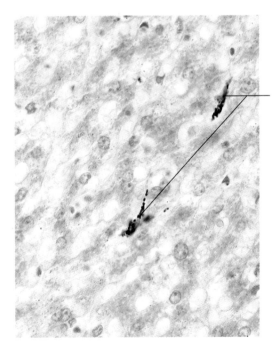

Kupffer cells
containing phagocytosed
Indian ink

Fig. 12-63. Section of **liver** in which the Kupffer cells have been stained vitally by the injection of Indian ink into the portal vein of the living animal prior to the preparation of the section (the section is counterstained with hematoxylin). x660.

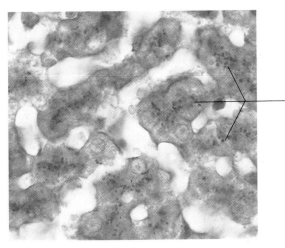

Glycogen granules

Fig. 12-64. Section of **liver** showing PAS stained glycogen granules in the cytoplasm of the liver cells. x660.

Bile canaliculi

Bile canaliculi

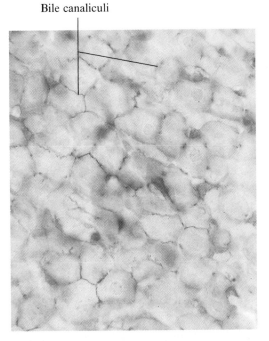

Fig. 12-65. Section of **liver** in which the bile canaliculi have been demonstrated by metal impregnation. Golgi staining. x440.

Fig. 12-66. Section of **liver** in which the bile canaliculi have been demonstrated by histochemical staining for adenosine triphosphatase. x440.

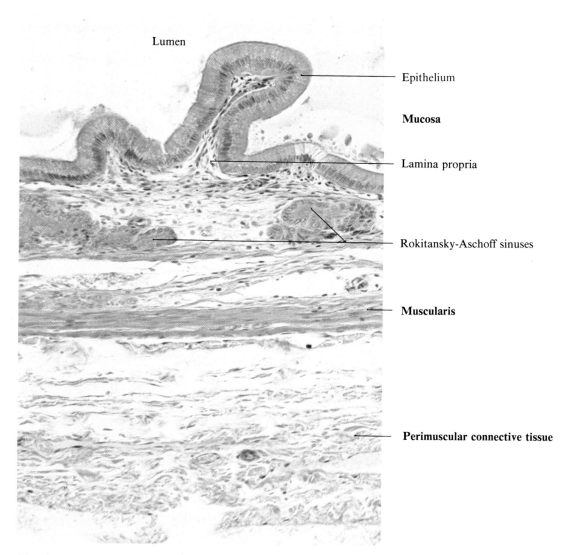

Lumen

Epithelium

Mucosa

Lamina propria

Rokitansky-Aschoff sinuses

Muscularis

Perimuscular connective tissue

Fig. 12-67. Part of the wall of the **gall bladder.** H and E. x220.

CHAPTER 13

The Respiratory System

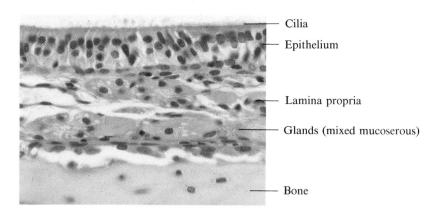

— Cilia
— Epithelium

— Lamina propria

— Glands (mixed mucoserous)

— Bone

Fig. 13-1. Part of the **nasal respiratory mucosa.** H and E. x440.

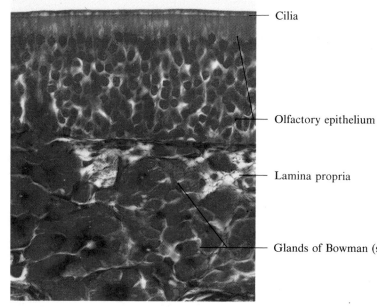

— Cilia

— Olfactory epithelium

— Lamina propria

— Glands of Bowman (serous)

Fig. 13-2. Part of the **olfactory mucosa** (the nasal mucosa of the olfactory region). Note the very tall epithelium and the thick lamina propria which is almost entirely occupied by the serous glands of Bowman. Azan. x440.

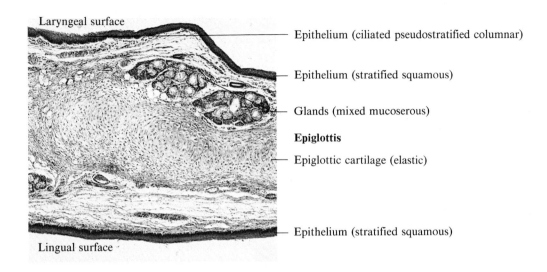

Laryngeal surface

Epithelium (ciliated pseudostratified columnar)

Epithelium (stratified squamous)

Glands (mixed mucoserous)

Epiglottis

Epiglottic cartilage (elastic)

Epithelium (stratified squamous)

Lingual surface

Fig. 13-3. Longitudinal section through part of the **epiglottis.** H and E. x55.

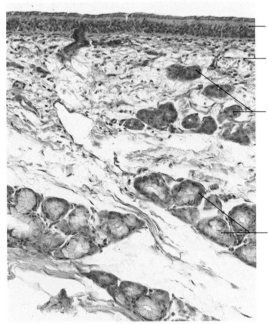

Epithelium

Lamina propria

Serous glands

Mixed mucoserous glands

Fig. 13-4. Part of the **laryngeal mucosa** in the part of the larynx which is lined with a ciliated pseudostratified columnar epithelium. H and E. x180.

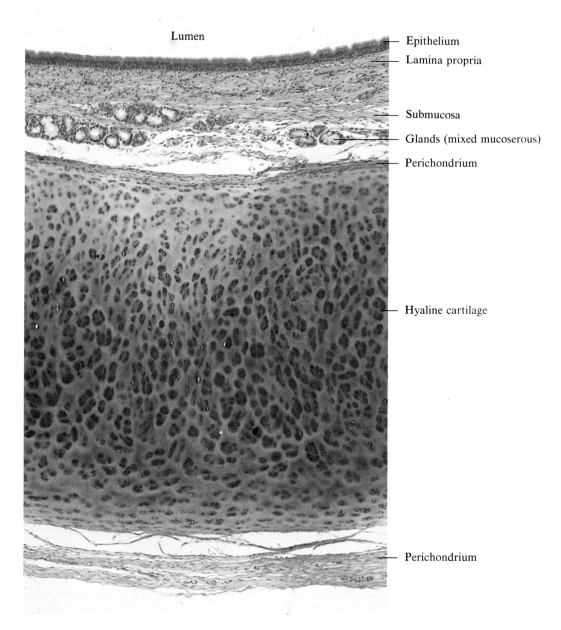

Lumen — Epithelium
— Lamina propria

— Submucosa
— Glands (mixed mucoserous)
— Perichondrium

— Hyaline cartilage

— Perichondrium

Fig. 13-5. Transverse section through the wall of the **trachea.** H and E. x90.

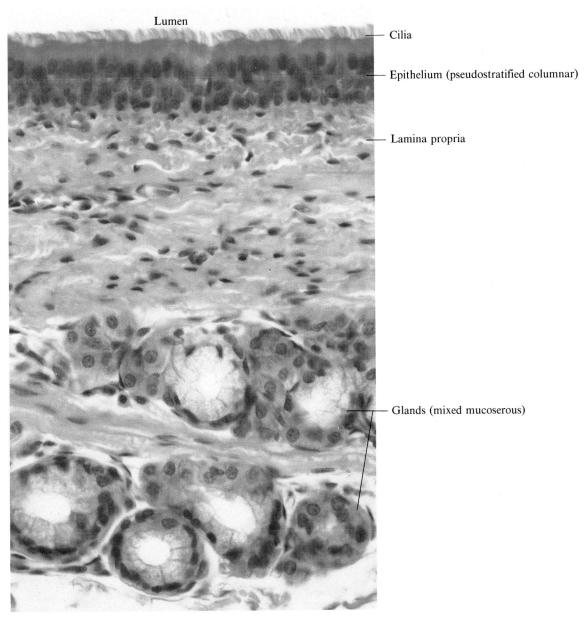

Lumen — Cilia

— Epithelium (pseudostratified columnar)

— Lamina propria

— Glands (mixed mucoserous)

Fig. 13-6. Part of the **mucosa of the trachea.** H and E. x505.

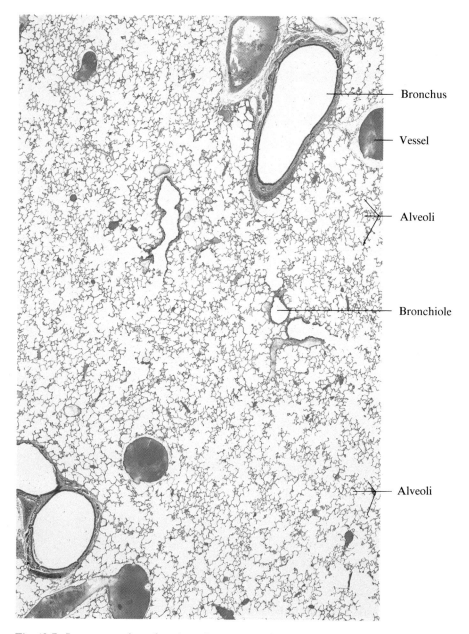

Fig. 13-7. Low power view of section of a **lung.** H and E. x17.

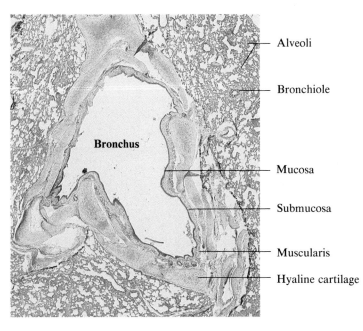

Alveoli

Bronchiole

Bronchus

Mucosa

Submucosa

Muscularis

Hyaline cartilage

Fig. 13-8. Cross sectional view of a large **bronchus.**
H and E. x14.

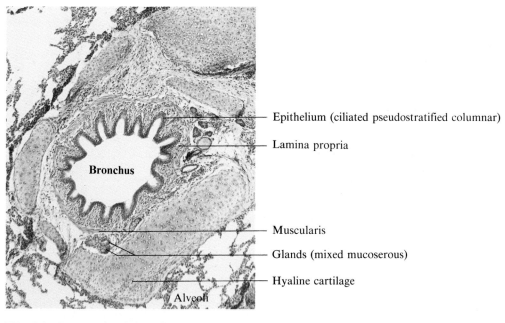

Epithelium (ciliated pseudostratified columnar)

Lamina propria

Bronchus

Muscularis

Glands (mixed mucoserous)

Hyaline cartilage

Alveoli

Fig. 13-9. Cross sectional view of a small **bronchus.**
H and E. x65.

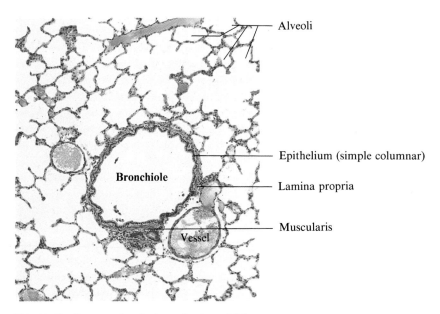

Fig. 13-10. Cross sectional view of a **bronchiole.**
Note that the pseudostratified columnar epithelium
now has been replaced by simple columnar epithelium and that cartilage and glands no longer are
present. H and E. x65.

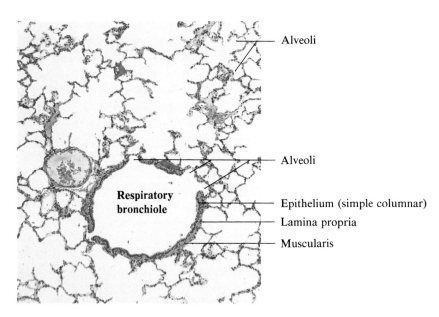

Fig. 13-11. Cross sectional view of a **respiratory
bronchiole.** Note the presence of alveoli in the
bronchiolar wall. H and E. x65.

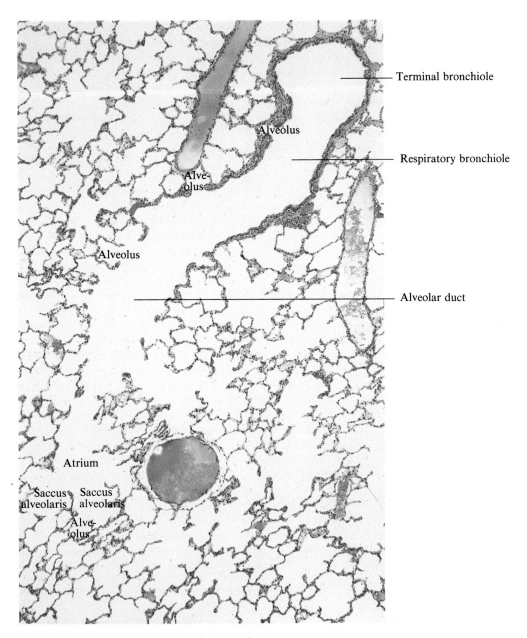

Terminal bronchiole

Respiratory bronchiole

Alveolar duct

Alveolus

Alve-
olus

Alveolus

Atrium

Saccus
alveolaris

Saccus
alveolaris

Alve-
olus

Fig. 13-12. Section of a **lung** showing the successive segments of the bronchial tree from a terminal bronchiole to the alveolar sacs. H and E. x65.

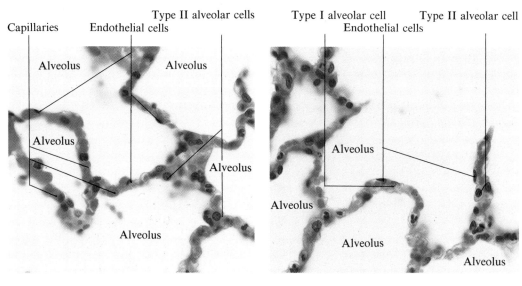

Fig. 13-13. High power view of a section of a **lung** showing alveolar walls. H and E. x440.

Fig. 13-14. High power view of a section of a **lung** showing alveolar walls. H and E. x440.

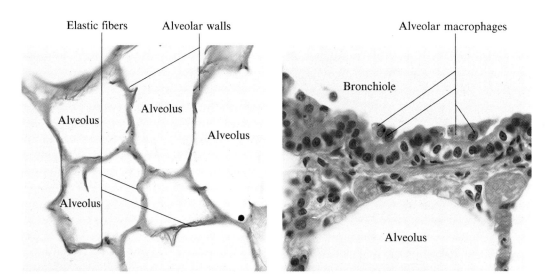

Fig. 13-15. High power view of an elastin stained section of a **lung.** Orcein staining. x275.

Fig. 13-16. Alveolar macrophages resting on the epithelium of a small **bronchiole**. Note the content of phagocytosed dust particles in the cytoplasm of the macrophages. H and E. x440.

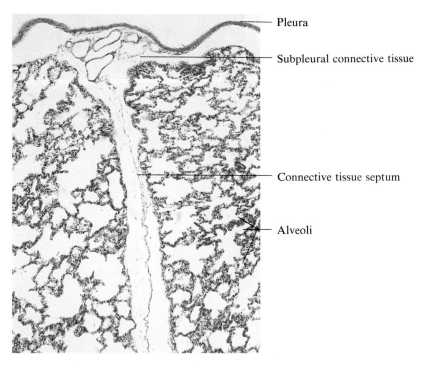

Pleura

Subpleural connective tissue

Connective tissue septum

Alveoli

Fig. 13-17. Section through the superficial part of the **lung.** H and E. x55.

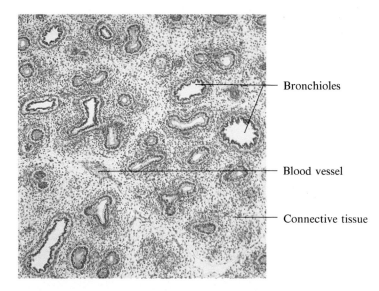

Bronchioles

Blood vessel

Connective tissue

Fig. 13-18. Part of an **embryonic lung** in the pseudoglandular period of development (from a human fetus in the 12th week of development). H and E. x65.

CHAPTER 14

The Urinary System

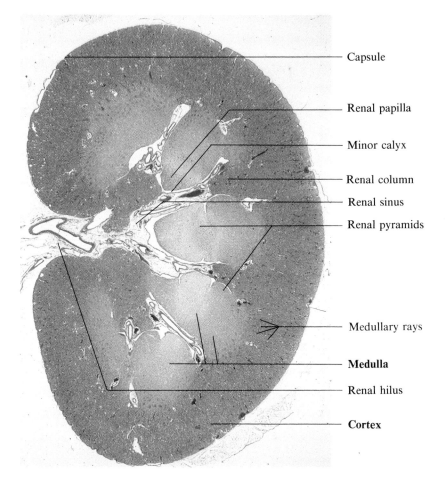

Capsule

Renal papilla

Minor calyx

Renal column

Renal sinus

Renal pyramids

Medullary rays

Medulla

Renal hilus

Cortex

Fig. 14-1. Low power view of a longitudinal section through the **kidney** of a cat. H and E. x4.

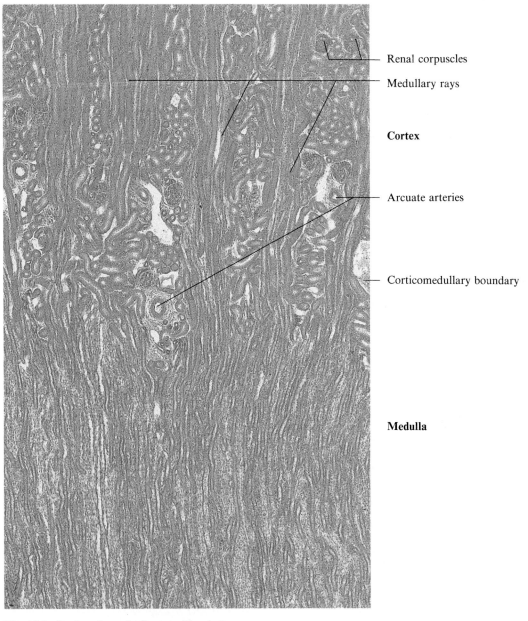

Renal corpuscles

Medullary rays

Cortex

Arcuate arteries

Corticomedullary boundary

Medulla

Fig. 14-2. Section through the transition between the cortex and medulla of a **kidney.** H and E. x65.

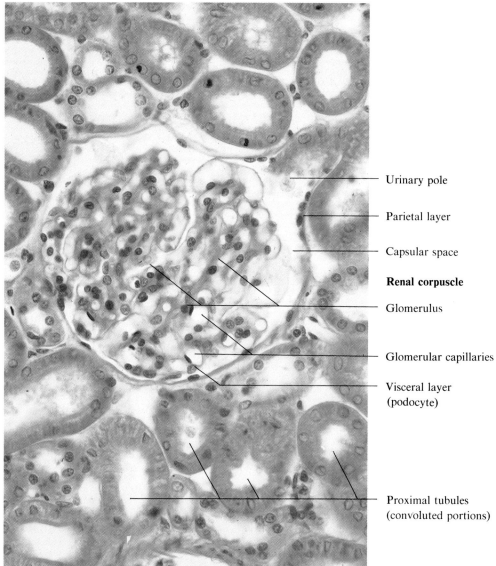

Urinary pole

Parietal layer

Capsular space

Renal corpuscle

Glomerulus

Glomerular capillaries

Visceral layer
(podocyte)

Proximal tubules
(convoluted portions)

Fig. 14-3. Section through part of the **renal cortex**
showing a renal corpuscle. H and E. x415.

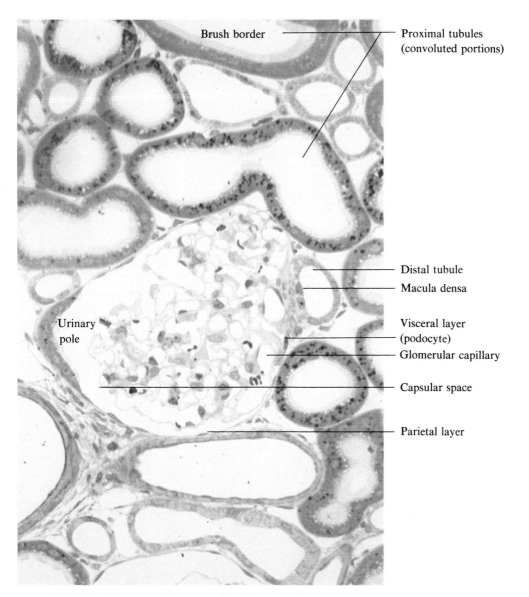

Brush border — Proximal tubules (convoluted portions)

Distal tubule
Macula densa

Visceral layer (podocyte)
Glomerular capillary

Capsular space

Parietal layer

Urinary pole

Fig. 14-4. Section through part of the **renal cortex** showing a renal corpuscle. Epon-embedded section stained with methylene blue. x400.

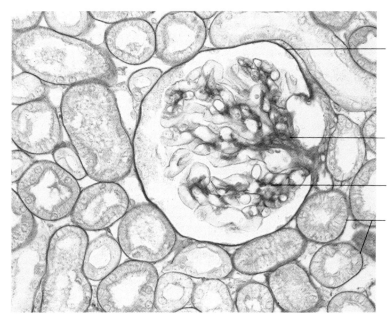

Basement membrane
of parietal layer

Mesangial matrix

Glomerular basement membrane

Basement membranes
of proximal tubules

Fig. 14-5. PAS stained section of the **renal cortex.**
The basement membranes are distinctly seen. PAS
staining. x325.

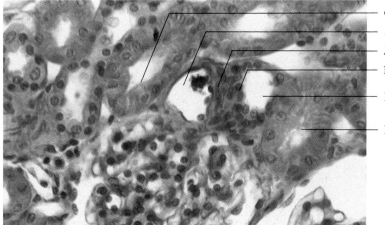

Collecting tubule
Afferent arteriole
Juxtaglomerular cells
Macula densa
Distal tubule
Proximal tubule

Fig. 14-6. Section through part of the **renal cortex.**
H and E. x400.

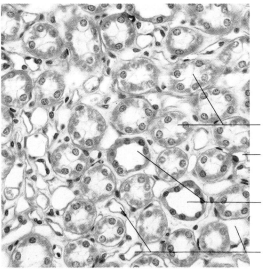

Fig. 14-7. Part of a cross section through the outer part of the **renal medulla.** H and E. x275.

Collecting tubules

Capillary

Ascending thick segments

Descending thin segments

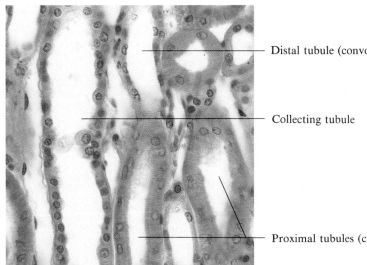

Fig. 14-8. Section through part of the **renal cortex.** H and E. x375.

Distal tubule (convoluted portion)

Collecting tubule

Proximal tubules (convoluted portions)

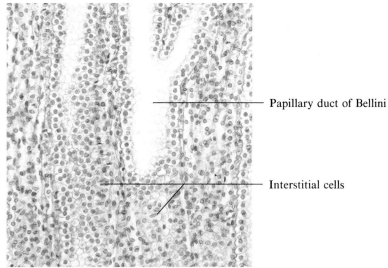

Papillary duct of Bellini

Interstitial cells

Fig. 14-9. Longitudinal section through the **renal medulla** just above the papilla. Note the characteristic appearance of the nuclei of the interstitial cells resembling the »rungs of a ladder«. H and E. x190.

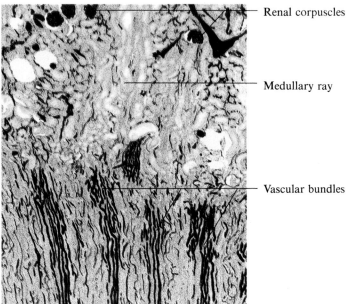

Renal corpuscles

Medullary ray

Vascular bundles

Fig. 14-10. Section of a **kidney** in which the renal artery was injected with Indian ink in the living animal before the preparation of the tissue section. x45.

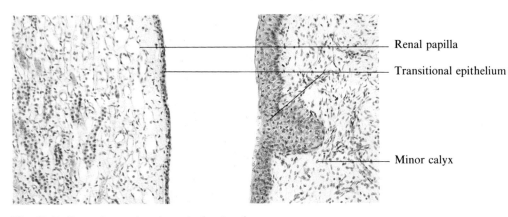

Renal papilla

Transitional epithelium

Minor calyx

Fig. 14-11. Part of a section through the tip of a **renal papilla** and the wall of the associated **minor calyx**. H and E. x110.

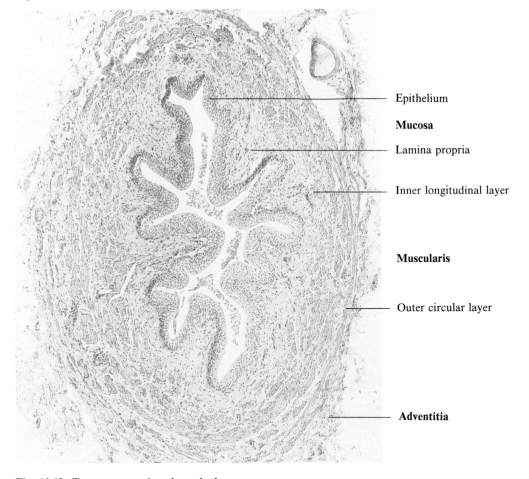

Epithelium

Mucosa

Lamina propria

Inner longitudinal layer

Muscularis

Outer circular layer

Adventitia

Fig. 14-12. Transverse section through the upper part of the **ureter.** H and E. x60.

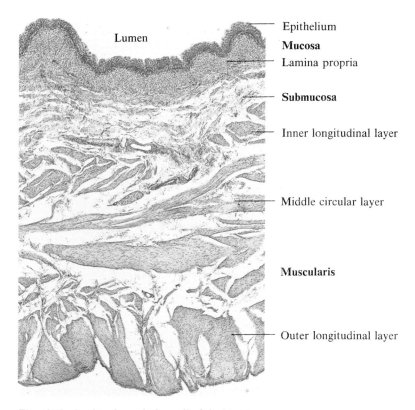

Epithelium
Mucosa
Lamina propria

Submucosa

Inner longitudinal layer

Middle circular layer

Muscularis

Outer longitudinal layer

Lumen

Fig. 14-13. Section through the wall of the **bladder** of a cat. Note the very thick muscularis. H and E. x75.

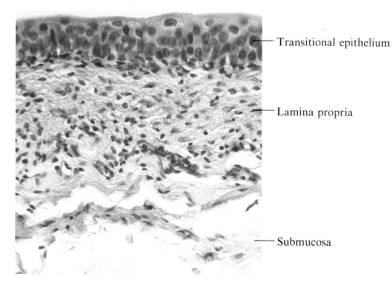

Transitional epithelium

Lamina propria

Submucosa

Fig. 14-14. Part of the **mucosa of the bladder.** H and E. x275.

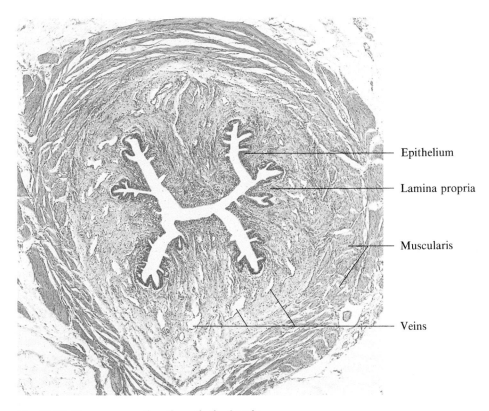

Fig. 14-15. Transverse section through the **female urethra.** Note the plexus of veins in the lamina propria. H and E. x45.

- Epithelium
- Lamina propria
- Muscularis
- Veins

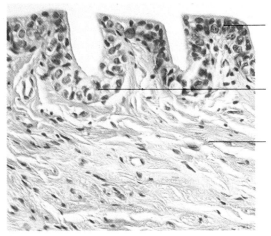

Fig. 14-16. High power view of the mucosa of the **female urethra** showing intraepithelial glands of Littré. H and E. x410.

- Transitional epithelium
- Intraepithelial gland of Littré
- Lamina propria

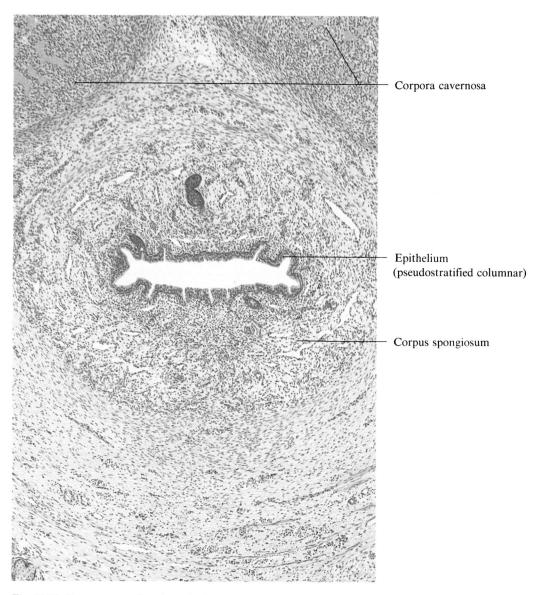

Corpora cavernosa

Epithelium
(pseudostratified columnar)

Corpus spongiosum

Fig. 14-17. Transverse section through the **spongy part of the male urethra.** H and E. x65.

CHAPTER 15

The Endocrine Glands

Connective tissue   Gland cells

Chromophobe   Sinusoids
Acidophils   Basophil

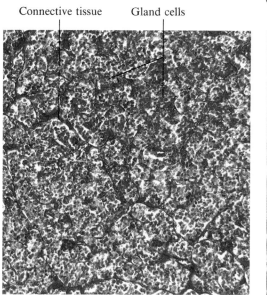

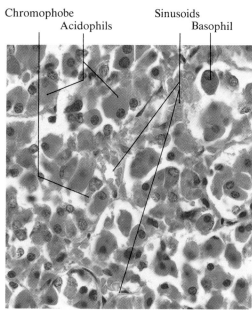

Fig. 15-1. Low power view of the **pars distalis of the hypophysis** showing the general histological structure. Azan. x65.

Fig. 15-2. High power view of the **pars distalis of the hypophysis.** H and E. x440.

Chromophobes
  Acidophils   Sinusoid   Basophils

Alpha cells (somatotropes)
           Sinusoids Basophils

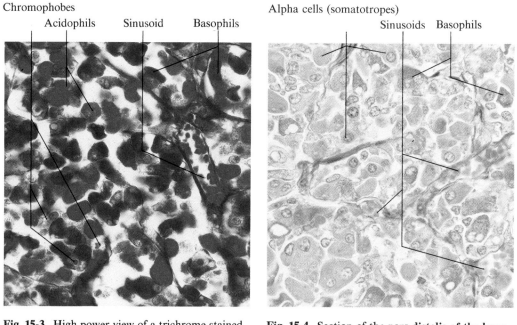

Fig. 15-3. High power view of a trichrome stained section of the **pars distalis of the hypophysis.** Note the sharper differentiation into acidophils and basophils with this staining (cp. Fig. 15-2). Azan. x440.

Fig. 15-4. Section of the **pars distalis of the hypophysis,** stained with the PAS reaction and orange G. The orangeophilic cells are alpha cells (Romeis' terminology) or somatotropes, whereas the PAS stained cells are beta cells. x440.

Gland cells

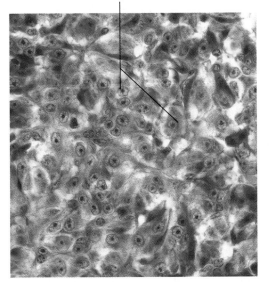

Portal venules   Parenchymal cells

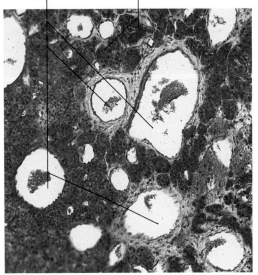

Fig. 15-5. Part of the **pars intermedia of the hypophysis.** Only one type of cell is seen which contains varying amounts of basophilic granules. Azan. x440.

Fig. 15-6. Horizontal section through the **pars tuberalis of the hypophysis.** Numerous portal venules are seen in cross sectional view, separated by clusters of epithelial parenchymal cells. Azan. x110.

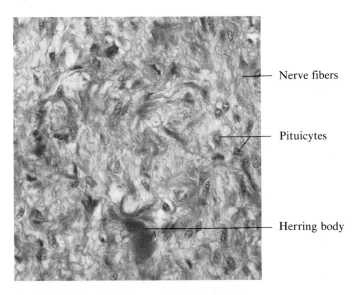

— Nerve fibers

— Pituicytes

— Herring body

Fig. 15-7. Part of the **pars nervosa of the hypophysis.** Azan. x440.

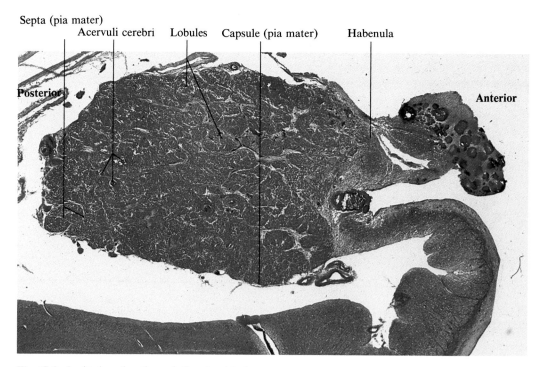

Fig. 15-8. Sagittal section through the **pineal body.**
Toluidine blue. x19.

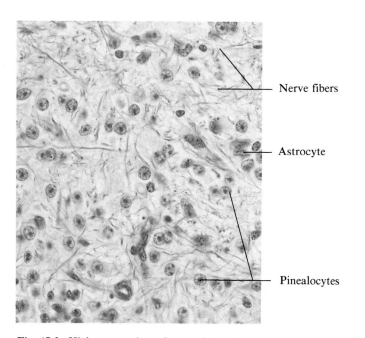

Fig. 15-9. High power view of part of the **pineal body.** Note the flattened nuclei of the astrocytes.
Azan. x440.

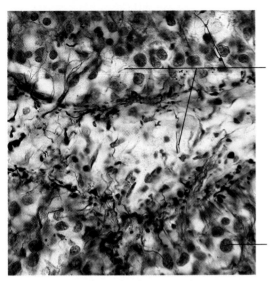

Nerve fibers

Pinealocyte

Fig. 15-10. Part of the **pineal body,** stained specifically for the demonstration of the nerve fibers. Bodian staining. x440.

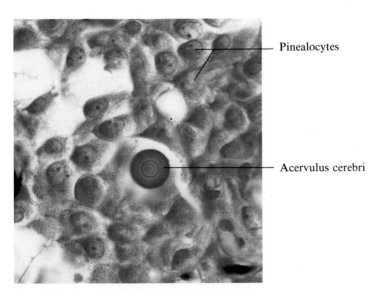

Pinealocytes

Acervulus cerebri

Fig. 15-11. Part of the **pineal body** showing an acervulus cerebri. Toluidine blue. x660.

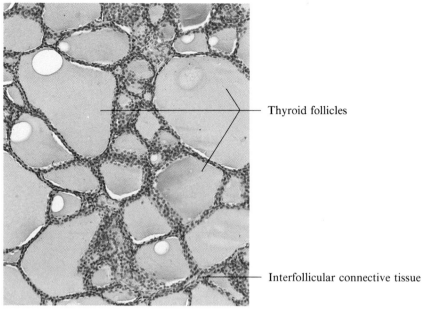

Thyroid follicles

Interfollicular connective tissue

Fig. 15-12. Part of the **thyroid gland.** Note the different sizes of the follicles. H and E. x110.

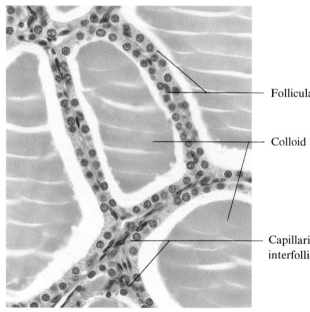

Follicular cells

Colloid in follicular lumen

Capillaries in interfollicular connective tissue

Fig. 15-13. High power view of part of the **thyroid gland.** Note the very sparse interfollicular connective tissue. H and E. x440.

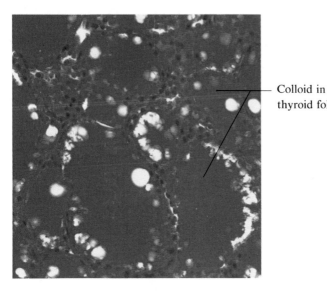

Colloid in
thyroid follicles

Fig. 15-14. PAS stained section of the **thyroid gland.** Note the intense staining of the colloid, which is a glycoprotein. PAS. x275.

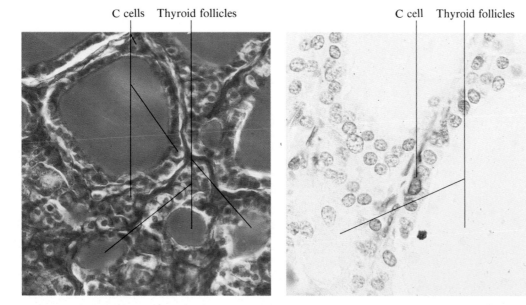

Fig. 15-15. Section of the **thyroid gland,** stained specifically for the demonstration of the C cells. Cajal's silver nitrate method. x340.

Fig. 15-16. Section of a **thyroid gland** in which the C cells are demonstrated immunohistochemically. x540.

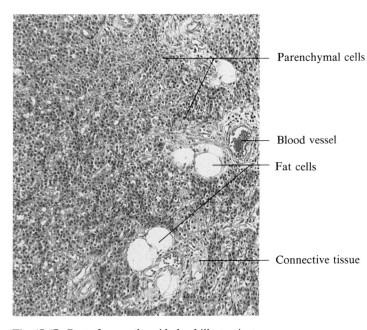

Parenchymal cells

Blood vessel

Fat cells

Connective tissue

Fig. 15-17. Part of a **parathyroid gland** illustrating the general histological structure. H and E. x135.

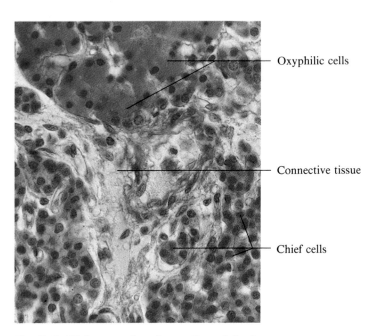

Oxyphilic cells

Connective tissue

Chief cells

Fig. 15-18. High power view of a **parathyroid gland** showing a group of oxyphilic cells. Azan. x440.

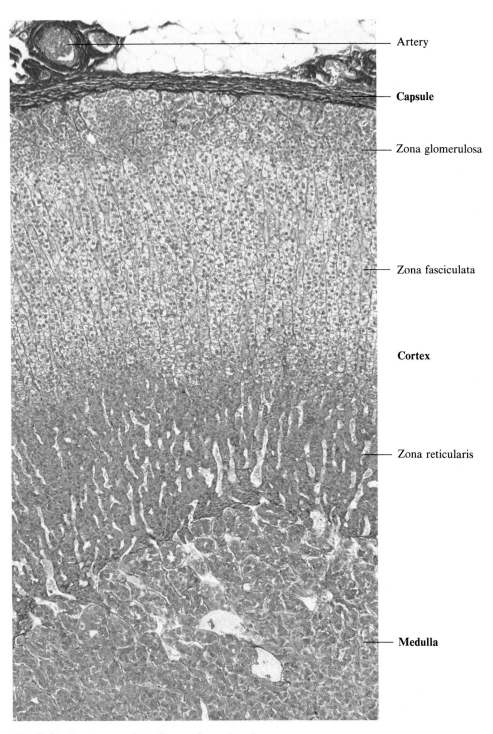

Artery

Capsule

Zona glomerulosa

Zona fasciculata

Cortex

Zona reticularis

Medulla

Fig. 15-19. Low power view of part of an **adrenal gland.** Azan. x110.

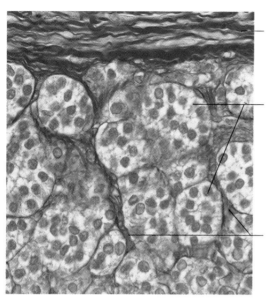

Capsule

Gland cells

Zona glomerulosa

Sinusoids

Fig. 15-20. Section through part of the **zona glomerulosa of an adrenal gland.** Azan. x440.

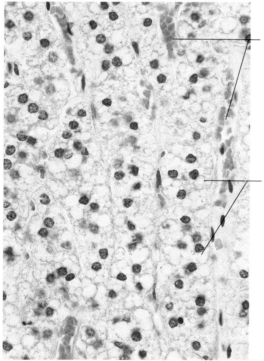

Sinusoids

Zona fasciculata

Spongiocytes

Fig. 15-21. Section through part of the **zona fasciculata of an adrenal gland.** The empty vacuoles in the spongiocytes are due to the extraction of lipid. H and E. x440.

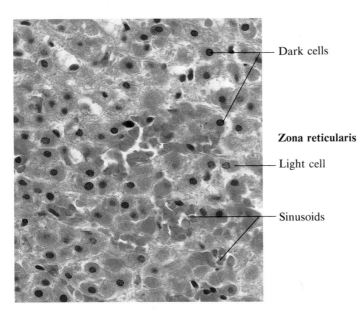

Dark cells

Zona reticularis

Light cell

Sinusoids

Fig. 15-22. Section through part of the **zona reticularis of an adrenal gland.** H and E. x440.

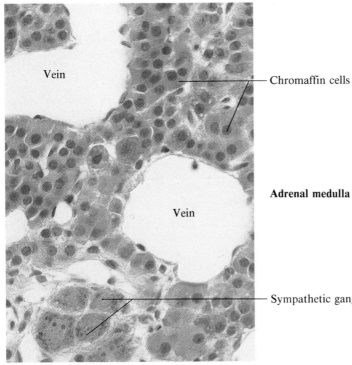

Vein

Chromaffin cells

Adrenal medulla

Vein

Sympathetic ganglion cells

Fig. 15-23. Part of the **adrenal medulla** showing slightly basophilic chromaffin cells and a cluster of sympathetic ganglion cells. Note the large, thin-walled veins. H and E. x440.

CHAPTER 16

The Reproductive System

Interstitial cells   Hilus   **Medulla**   **Cortex**   Tunica albuginea

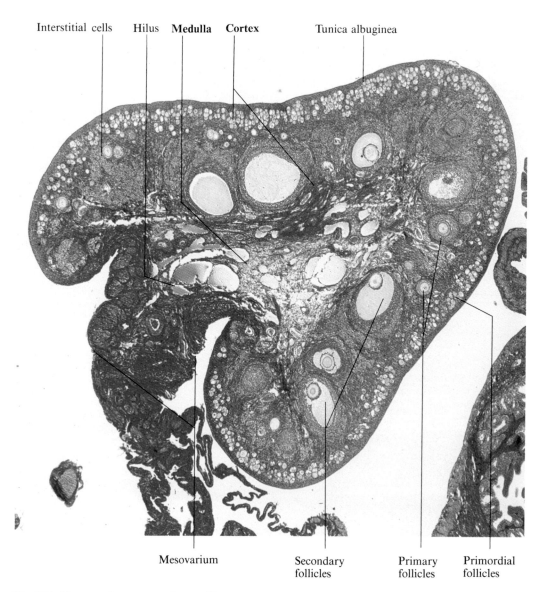

Mesovarium   Secondary   Primary   Primordial
                    follicles   follicles   follicles

Fig. 16-1. Transected cat **ovary.** Azan. x29.

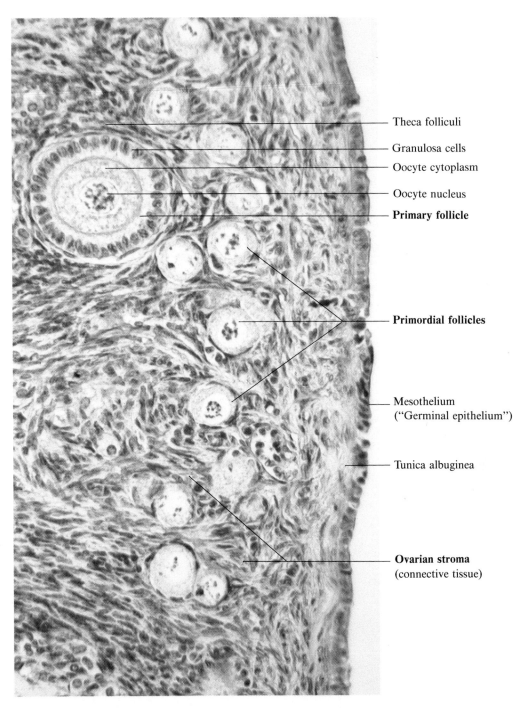

Theca folliculi

Granulosa cells

Oocyte cytoplasm

Oocyte nucleus

Primary follicle

Primordial follicles

Mesothelium
("Germinal epithelium")

Tunica albuginea

Ovarian stroma
(connective tissue)

Fig. 16-2. Section through the superficial part of
the **ovary.** H and E. x400.

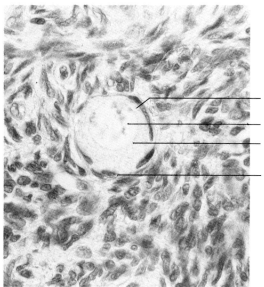

Cytoplasm

Oocyte

Nucleus

Oocyte

Primordial follicle

Follicular cell

Fig. 16-3. Primordial follicle in the **cortex of the ovary.** H and E. x680.

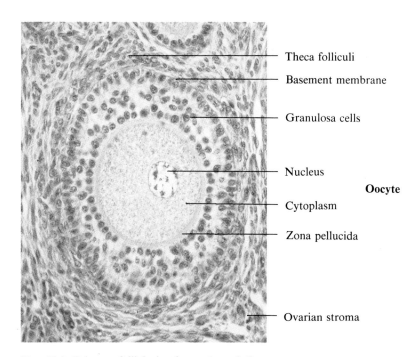

Theca folliculi

Basement membrane

Granulosa cells

Nucleus

Oocyte

Cytoplasm

Zona pellucida

Ovarian stroma

Fig. 16-4. Primary follicle in the **cortex of the ovary.** H and E. x275.

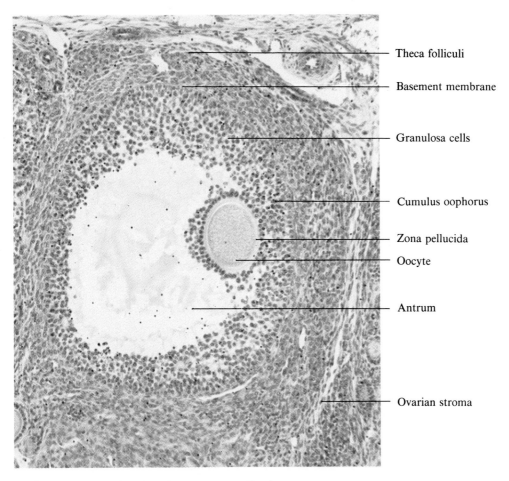

Theca folliculi

Basement membrane

Granulosa cells

Cumulus oophorus

Zona pellucida

Oocyte

Antrum

Ovarian stroma

Fig. 16-5. Secondary follicle in the **ovary.** H and E.
x150.

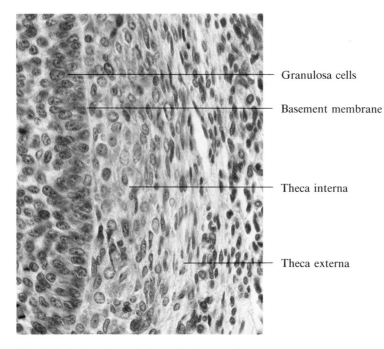

Granulosa cells

Basement membrane

Theca interna

Theca externa

Fig. 16-6. Section through the wall of a secondary follicle in the **ovary.** H and E. x440.

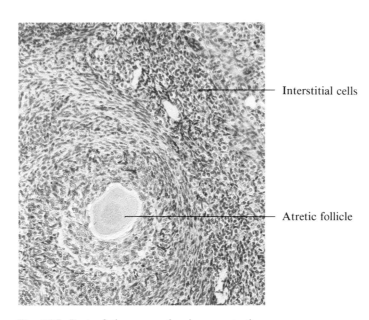

Interstitial cells

Atretic follicle

Fig. 16-7. Part of the **ovary** showing an atretic follicle and interstitial cells. H and E. x135.

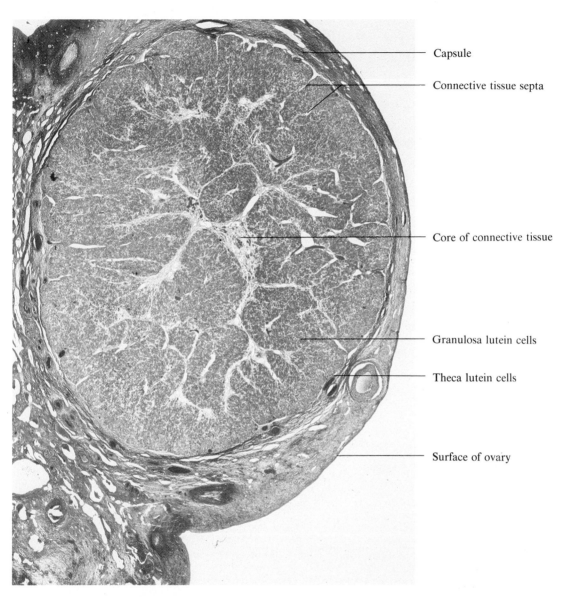

Capsule

Connective tissue septa

Core of connective tissue

Granulosa lutein cells

Theca lutein cells

Surface of ovary

Fig. 16-8. Transected **corpus luteum.** Azan. x13.

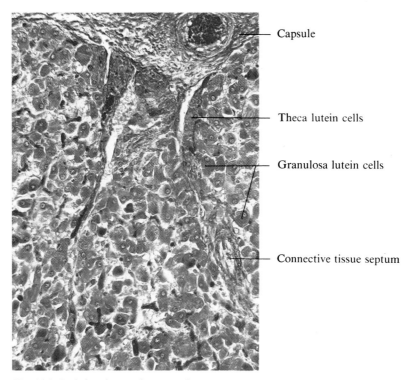

Capsule

Theca lutein cells

Granulosa lutein cells

Connective tissue septum

Fig. 16-9. Peripheral part of a **corpus luteum.** Azan. x135.

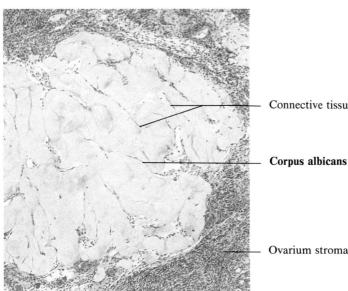

Connective tissue cords

Corpus albicans

Ovarium stroma

Fig. 16-10. Part of a **corpus albicans.** H and E. x65.

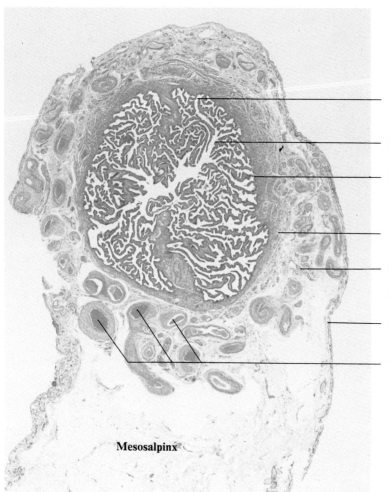

Epithelium

Mucosa

Lamina propria

Inner circular layer

Muscularis

Outer longitudinal layer

Submesothelial connective tissue

Serosa (peritoneum)

Mesothelium

Vessels

Mesosalpinx

Fig. 16-11. Transverse section through the **ampulla of the uterine (Fallopian) tube.** Note the characteristic labyrinthine lumen due to the large number of branched, longitudinal folds of the mucosa. H and E. x14.

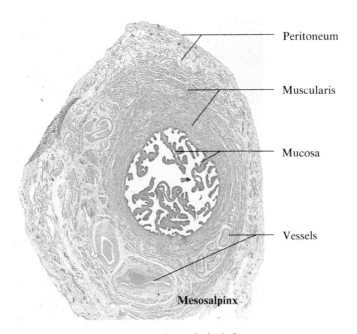

Peritoneum

Muscularis

Mucosa

Vessels

Mesosalpinx

Fig. 16-12. Transverse section through the **isthmus of the uterine (Fallopian) tube.** Note the smaller lumen with fewer mucosal folds than in the ampulla (compare with Fig. 16-11) as well as the thicker circular muscle layer. H and E. x18.

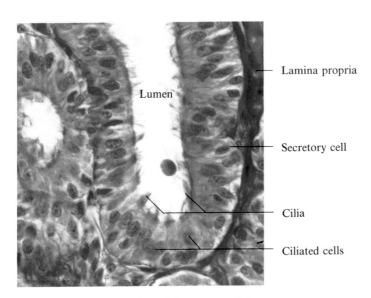

Lamina propria

Lumen

Secretory cell

Cilia

Ciliated cells

Fig. 16-13. High power view of the **mucosa of the uterine (Fallopian) tube.** Azan. x440.

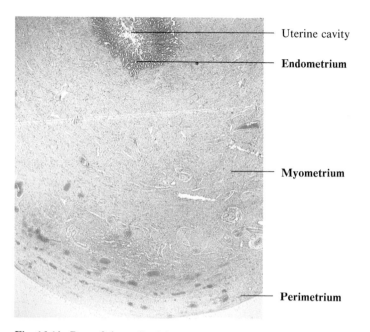

Uterine cavity

Endometrium

Myometrium

Perimetrium

Fig. 16-14. Part of the wall of the **uterine body.** H and E. x5.

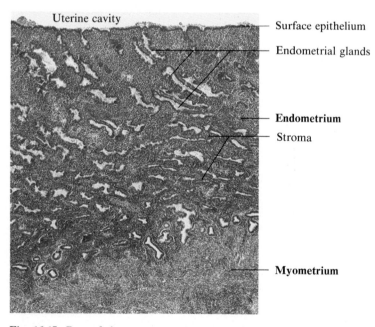

Uterine cavity

Surface epithelium

Endometrial glands

Endometrium

Stroma

Myometrium

Fig. 16-15. Part of the **mucosa (endometrium) of the uterine body.** H and E. x35.

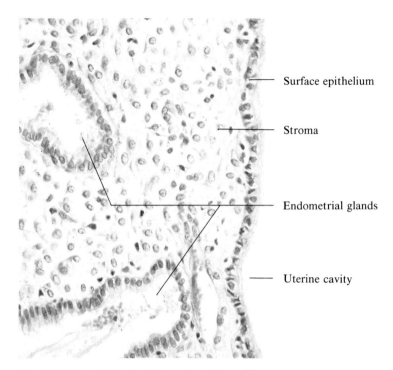

Surface epithelium

Stroma

Endometrial glands

Uterine cavity

Fig. 16-16. Luminal part of the **endometrium** with surface epithelium. H and E. x275.

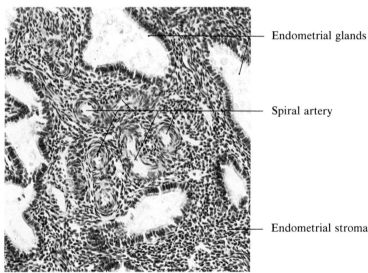

Endometrial glands

Spiral artery

Endometrial stroma

Fig. 16-17. Spiral artery in the **endometrium.** Note the numerous cross sectional profiles which result from the pronounced coiling of the spiral artery. H and E. x150.

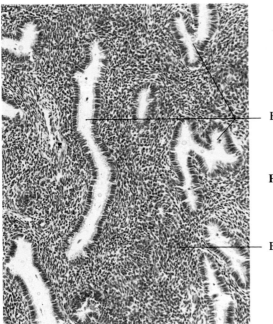

Endometrial glands

Proliferative phase

Endometrial stroma

Fig. 16-18. Endometrium in the **proliferative phase** of the menstrual cycle. H and E. x120.

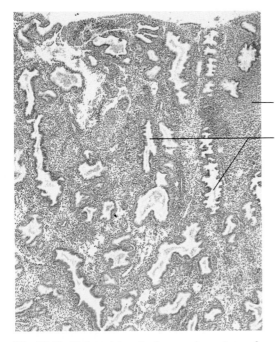

Endometrial stroma
Secretory phase
Endometrial glands

Fig. 16-19. Endometrium in the **secretory phase** of the menstrual cycle. Note the serrated glands with dilated lumen containing secretion. H and E. x45.

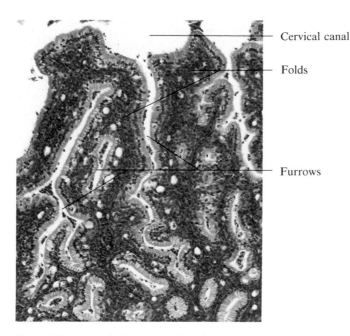

Cervical canal

Folds

Furrows

Fig. 16-20. Part of the endocervix, that is, the **mucosa of the uterine cervix.** H and E. x110.

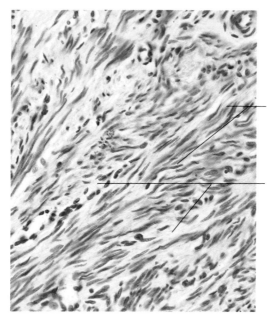

Smooth muscle cells

Myometrium

Connective tissue septa

Fig. 16-21. Section of the **myometrium of the uterine body.** Note the characteristic whirls formed by the bundles of smooth muscle cells. H and E. x275.

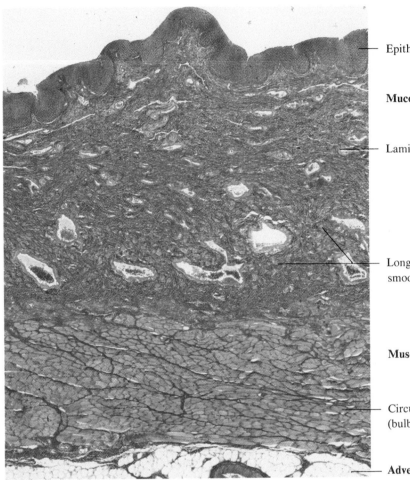

— Epithelium

Mucosa

— Lamina propria

— Longitudinal
smooth muscle

Muscularis

— Circular skeletal muscle
(bulbospongiosus)

— **Adventitia**

Fig. 16-22. Part of a cross section through the wall
of the **vagina.** Azan. x27.

Acidophilic cells

Clusters of navicular cells

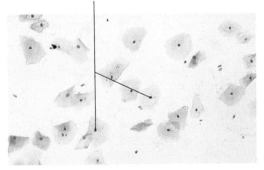

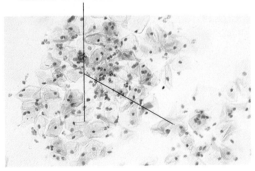

Fig. 16-23. Vaginal smear from the **late follicular
phase** of the menstrual cycle. Papanicolaou. x110.

Fig. 16-24. Vaginal smear from the **luteal phase** of
the menstrual cycle. Papanicolaou. x110.

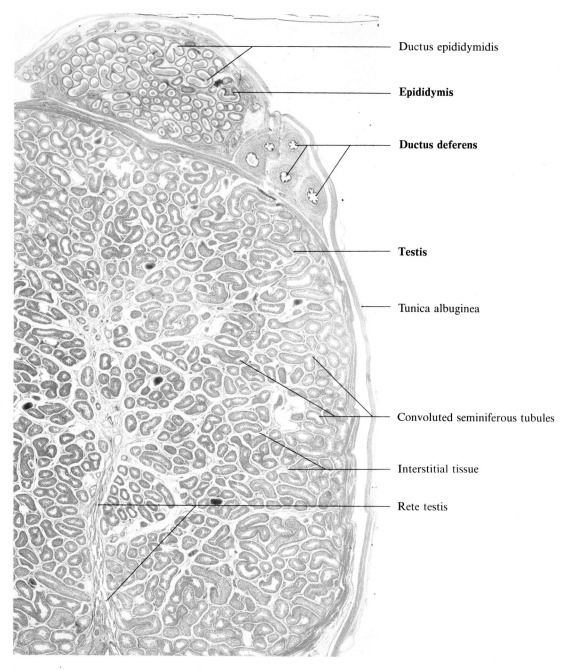

Ductus epididymidis

Epididymis

Ductus deferens

Testis

Tunica albuginea

Convoluted seminiferous tubules

Interstitial tissue

Rete testis

Fig. 16-25. Section through part of the **testis,** the **epididymis** and the first, coiled portion of the **ductus deferens**. H and E. x13.

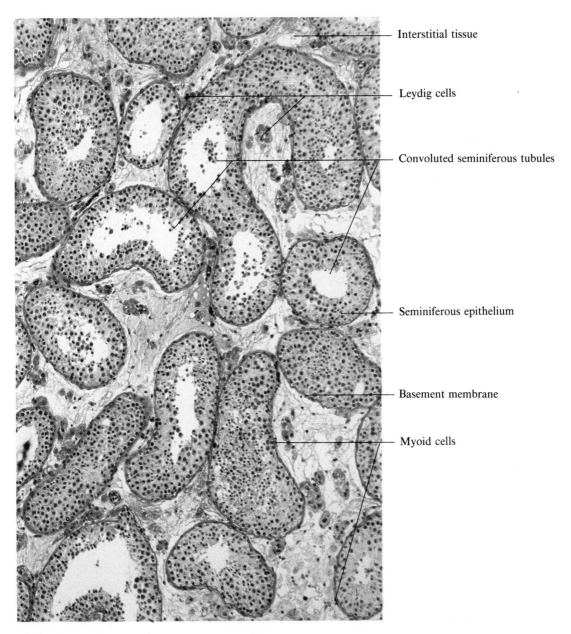

Interstitial tissue

Leydig cells

Convoluted seminiferous tubules

Seminiferous epithelium

Basement membrane

Myoid cells

Fig. 16-26. Section through part of the **testis.** H and E. x110.

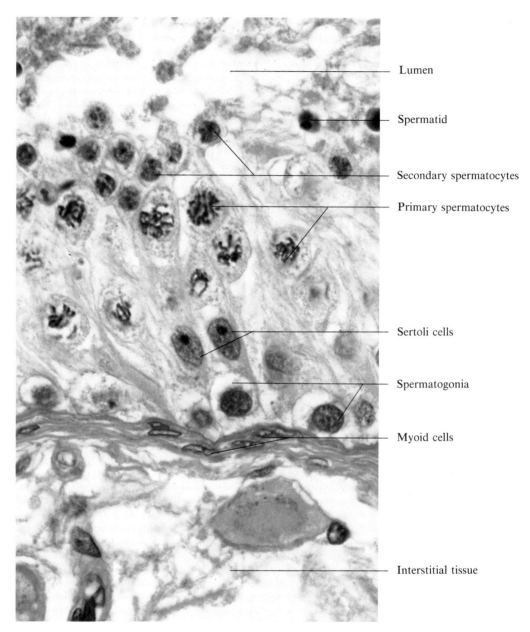

Lumen

Spermatid

Secondary spermatocytes

Primary spermatocytes

Sertoli cells

Spermatogonia

Myoid cells

Interstitial tissue

Fig. 16-27. High power view of a cross-sectioned, **coiled seminiferous tubule of the testis** showing the seminiferous epithelium. H and E. x1100.

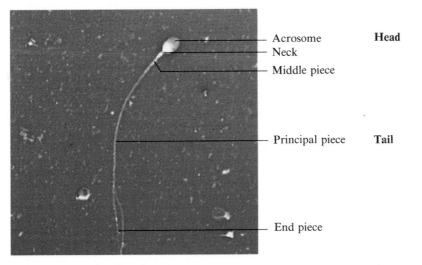

Acrosome — **Head**
Neck
Middle piece

Principal piece — **Tail**

End piece

Fig. 16-28. Smear of an ejaculate showing a human **spermatozoon.** H and E. (modified). x1100.

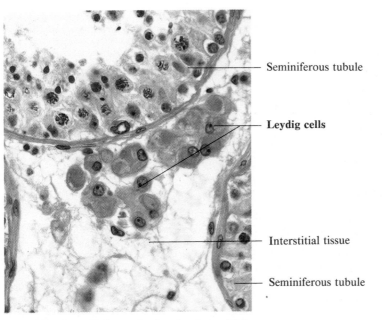

— Seminiferous tubule

— **Leydig cells**

— Interstitial tissue

— Seminiferous tubule

Fig. 16-29. Part of the **testis** showing interstitial tissue with clusters of Leydig cells. H and E. x440.

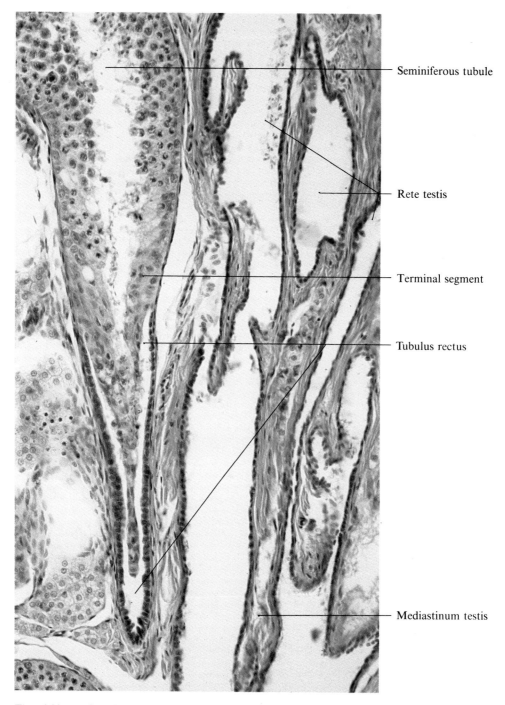

Seminiferous tubule

Rete testis

Terminal segment

Tubulus rectus

Mediastinum testis

Fig. 16-30. Section of the **testis** showing the transition of a seminiferous tubule into the tubulus rectus. In addition, part of the mediastinum testis with the rete testis is seen. H and E. x90.

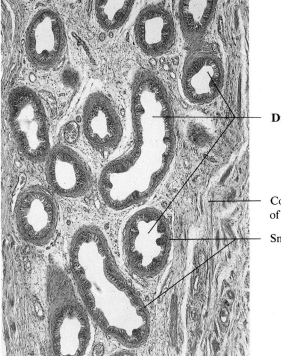
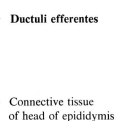

Ductuli efferentes

Connective tissue
of head of epididymis

Smooth muscle cells

Fig. 16-31. Section through the **head of the epididymis** showing several transected ductuli efferentes. Note the characteristic festooned luminal border of their epithelium. H and E. x110.

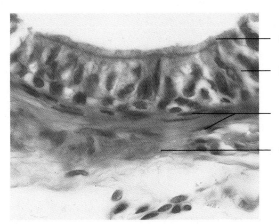

Cilia

Epithelium

Smooth muscle cells

Connective tissue

Fig. 16-32. Section through the **head of the epididymis** showing the mucosa of a ductulus efferens. H and E. x540.

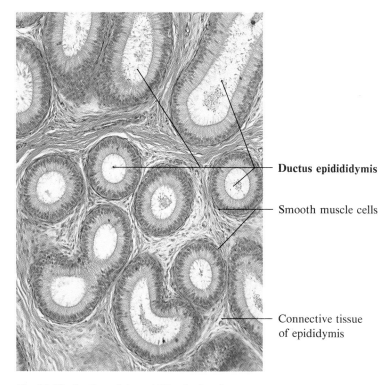

Ductus epidididymis

Smooth muscle cells

Connective tissue
of epididymis

Fig. 16-33. Section of the **epididymis** showing several cross sections of the ductus epididymidis. Note the very tall pseudostratified columnar epithelium with stereocilia. H and E. x110.

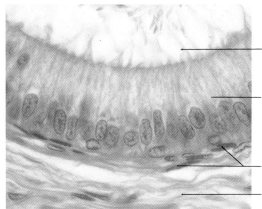

Stereocilia

Epithelium

Smooth muscle cells

Connective tissue

Fig. 16-34. Section of the **epididymis** showing the epithelium of the ductus epididymidis. H and E. x660.

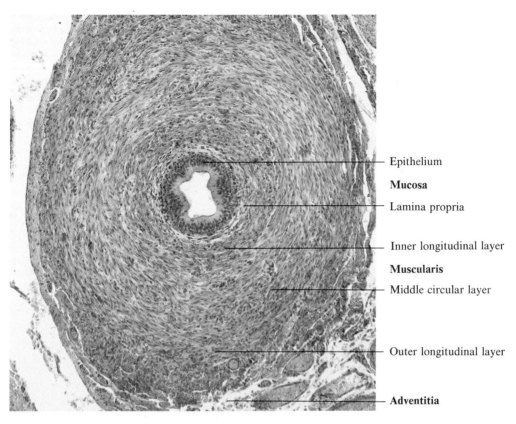

Epithelium

Mucosa

Lamina propria

Inner longitudinal layer

Muscularis

Middle circular layer

Outer longitudinal layer

Adventitia

Fig. 16-35. Cross section of the **ductus deferens.**
Note the highly developed muscularis. H and E.
x100.

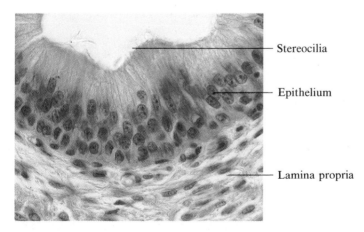

Stereocilia

Epithelium

Lamina propria

Fig. 16-36. Part of a cross sectioned **ductus deferens** showing the mucosa. H and E. x540.

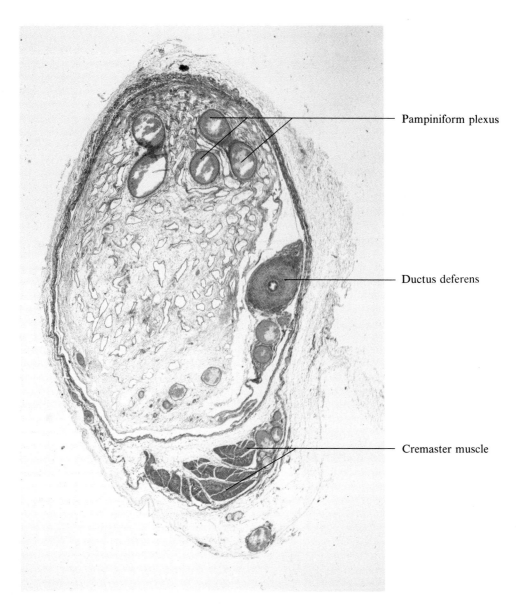

Pampiniform plexus

Ductus deferens

Cremaster muscle

Fig. 16-37. Cross section through the **spermatic cord.** H and E. x17.

Secretion in lumen   Mucosa   Muscularis   Adventitia

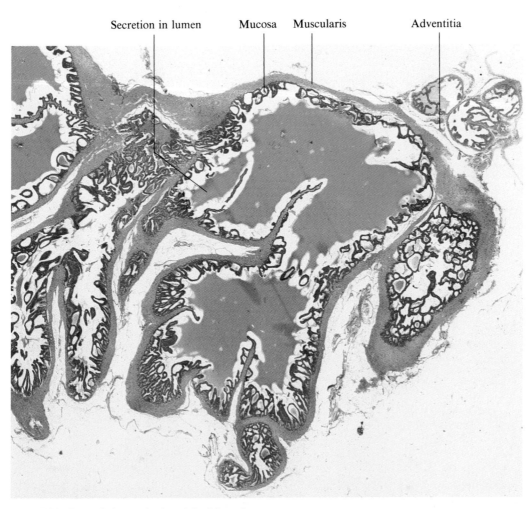

Fig. 16-38. Part of the **seminal vesicle.** Note the branched, anastomosing folds of the mucosa giving rise to apparently isolated cavities, all of which are, however, in continuity in the intact organ. H and E. x23.

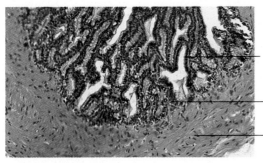

— Epithelium

— Lamina propria

— Muscularis

Fig. 16-39. Part of the **seminal vesicle** showing the mucosa. H and E. x110.

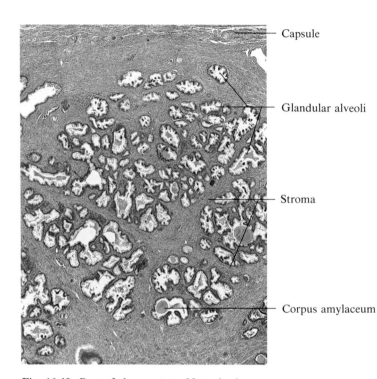

Capsule

Glandular alveoli

Stroma

Corpus amylaceum

Fig. 16-40. Part of the **prostate.** Note the large, irregularly shaped glandular alveoli of varying size, some of which contain corpora amylacea. H and E. x22.

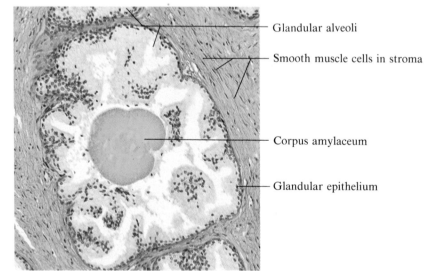

Glandular alveoli

Smooth muscle cells in stroma

Corpus amylaceum

Glandular epithelium

Fig. 16-41. Section of the **prostate** showing the glandular epithelium and a corpus amylaceum. Note the smooth muscle cells in the stroma. Van Gieson. x110.

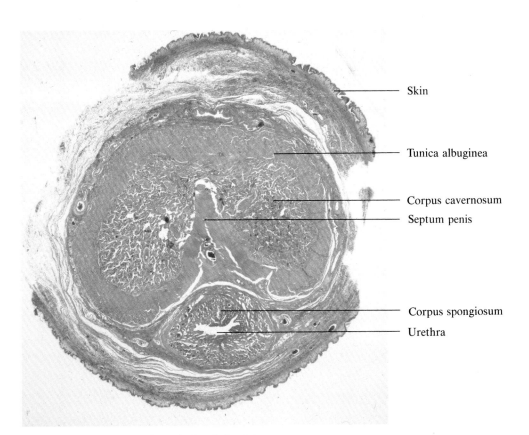

Skin

Tunica albuginea

Corpus cavernosum
Septum penis

Corpus spongiosum
Urethra

Fig. 16-42. Cross section through the shaft of the **penis.** H and E. x4.

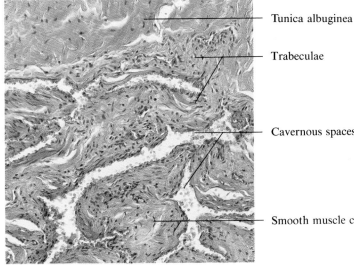

Tunica albuginea

Trabeculae

Cavernous spaces

Smooth muscle cells

Fig. 16-43. Part of a **corpus cavernosum penis.** Note the smooth muscle cells in the connective tissue trabecula separating the cavernous spaces. H and E. x110.

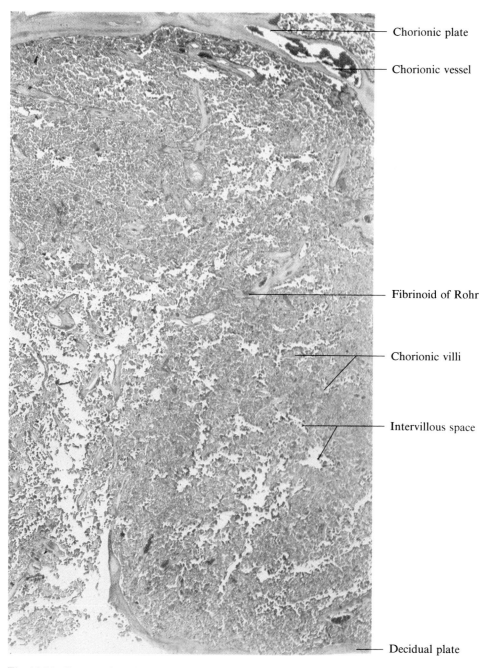

Chorionic plate

Chorionic vessel

Fibrinoid of Rohr

Chorionic villi

Intervillous space

Decidual plate

Fig. 16-44. Cross section of a full-term **placenta.** H and E. x10.

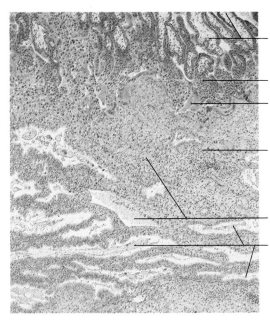

Chorionic villi

Anchoring villus

Invading syncytiotrophoblast

Decidua basalis

Uterine venous sinusoids

Uterine glands

Fig. 16-45. Endometrium at about 21 days of gestational age. The implantation site, with the tips of the chorionic villi belonging to the developing **placenta,** is seen in the upper part of the picture. H and E. x45.

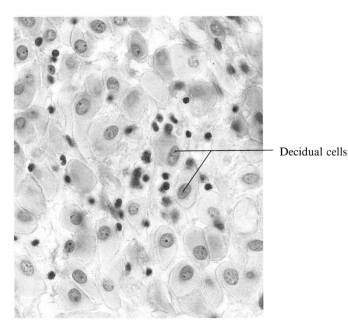

Decidual cells

Fig. 16-46. Decidual cells in the **endometrium** at about 21 days of gestational age. H and E. x440.

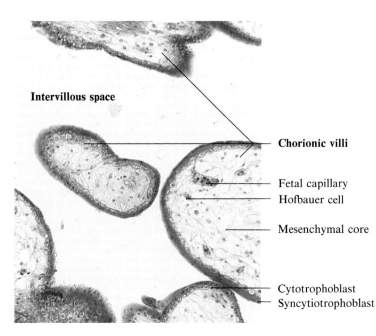

Intervillous space

Chorionic villi

Fetal capillary

Hofbauer cell

Mesenchymal core

Cytotrophoblast
Syncytiotrophoblast

Fig. 16-47. Chorionic villi from an early human **placenta.** Note the two layers of trophoblast. Azan. x110.

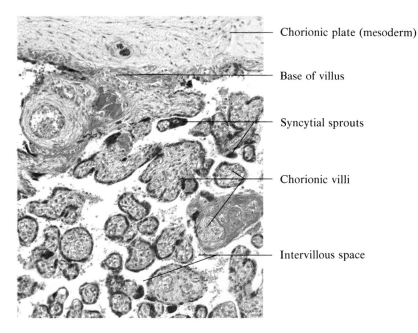

Chorionic plate (mesoderm)

Base of villus

Syncytial sprouts

Chorionic villi

Intervillous space

Fig. 16-48. Section of a full-term **placenta** near the basal plate showing several cross sectioned chorionic villi. H and E. x110.

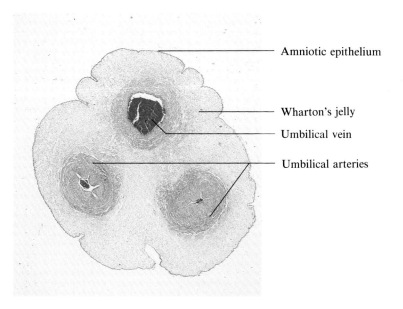

Amniotic epithelium

Wharton's jelly

Umbilical vein

Umbilical arteries

Fig. 16-49. Transverse section through the **umbilical cord** at full-term. H and E. x9.

CHAPTER 17

The Mammary Glands

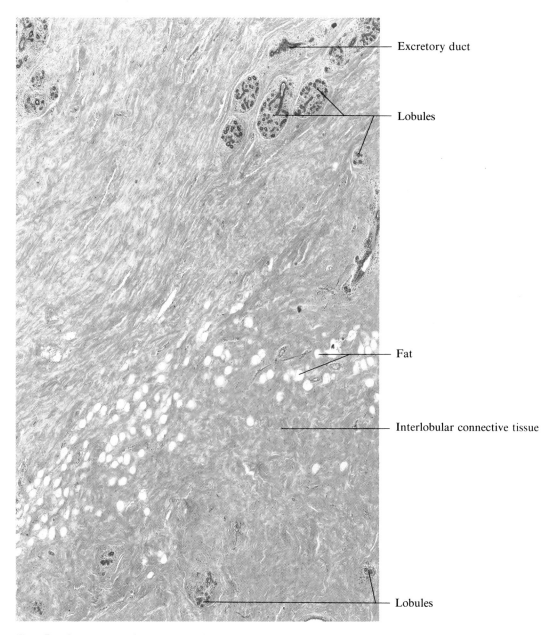

Excretory duct

Lobules

Fat

Interlobular connective tissue

Lobules

Fig. 17-1. Low power view of part of a **resting mammary gland.** Note the abundant interlobular connective tissue and the scattered lobules containing glandular tissue. H and E. x30.

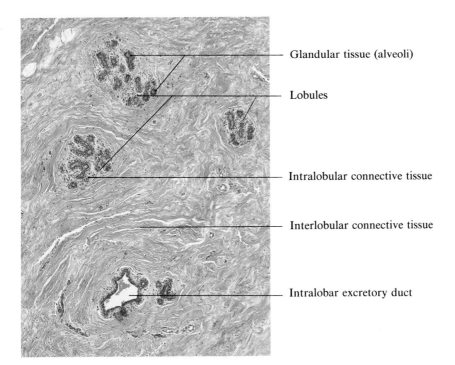

Glandular tissue (alveoli)

Lobules

Intralobular connective tissue

Interlobular connective tissue

Intralobar excretory duct

Fig. 17-2. Part of a lobe of a **resting mammary gland.** H and E. x55.

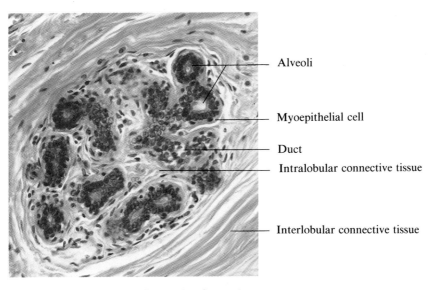

Alveoli

Myoepithelial cell

Duct
Intralobular connective tissue

Interlobular connective tissue

Fig. 17-3. Close up view of a lobule of a **resting mammary gland.** Note the cell-rich, loose intralobular connective tissue, as compared to the fibrous interlobular connective tissue. H and E. x240.

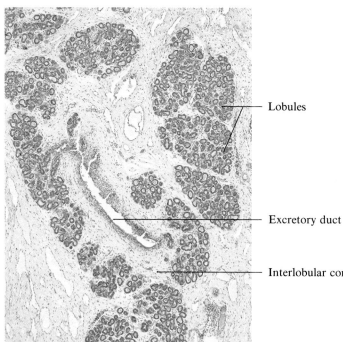

Lobules

Excretory duct

Interlobular connective tissue

Fig. 17-4. Part of a lobe of a **mammary gland from a pregnant woman.** Note the increased amount of glandular tissue which almost entirely fills the lobules. H and E. x45.

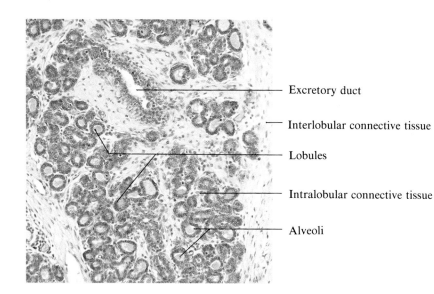

Excretory duct

Interlobular connective tissue

Lobules

Intralobular connective tissue

Alveoli

Fig. 17-5. Part of a **mammary gland from a pregnant woman,** seen at higher power. H and E. x110.

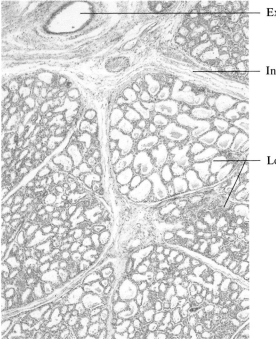

Excretory duct

Interlobular connective tissue

Lobules

Fig. 17-6. Part of a lobe of a **lactating mammary gland.** Note the different sizes of the alveoli. Also, note the very sparse intra- and interlobular connective tissue which almost entirely has been replaced by glandular tissue. H and E. x45.

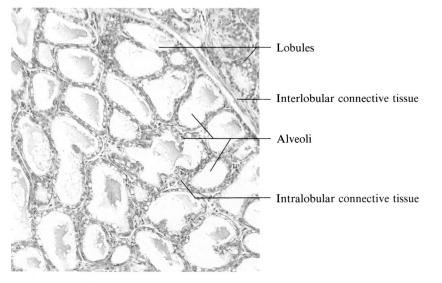

Lobules

Interlobular connective tissue

Alveoli

Intralobular connective tissue

Fig. 17-7. Part of a **lactating mammary gland,** seen at higher power. H and E. x110.

CHAPTER 18

The Eye

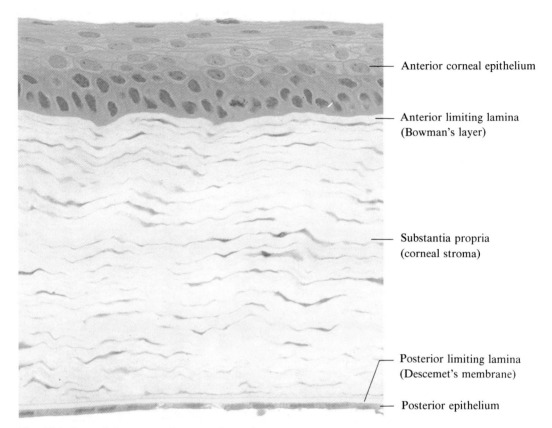

Anterior corneal epithelium

Anterior limiting lamina
(Bowman's layer)

Substantia propria
(corneal stroma)

Posterior limiting lamina
(Descemet's membrane)

Posterior epithelium

Fig. 18-1. Part of the **cornea** from a guinea pig
(Bowman's layer is very thin). Hematoxylin and
eosin stained metachrylate-embedded section.
x505.

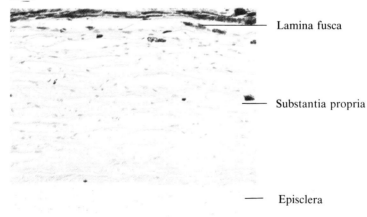

Lamina fusca

Substantia propria

Episclera

Fig. 18-2. Part of a meridional section through the
sclera. H and E. x145.

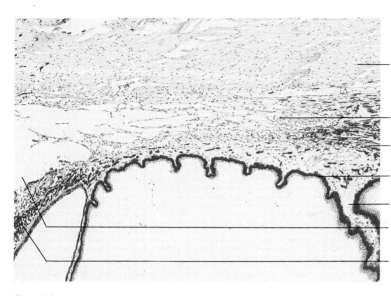

Fig. 18-3. Meridional section through the **limbus of the eye** showing the iridocorneal angle and the trabecular meshwork. H and E. x60.

Limbal (corneoscleral) stroma

Trabecular meshwork

Ciliary muscle

Ciliary epithelium

Ciliary proces

Iridocorneal angle

Iris

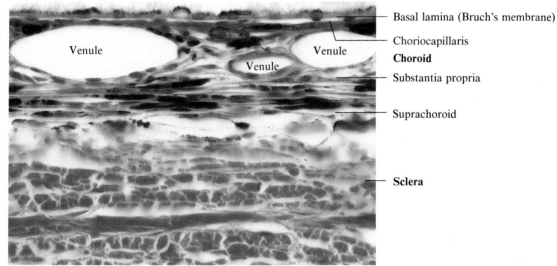

Basal lamina (Bruch's membrane)

Choriocapillaris

Choroid

Substantia propria

Suprachoroid

Sclera

Venule

Venule

Venule

Fig. 18-4. Part of a meridional section through the **choroid.** Azan. x440.

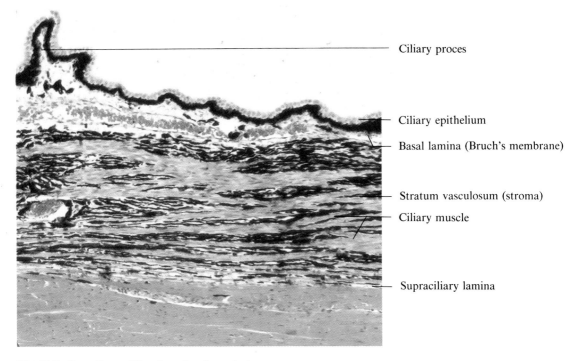

Ciliary proces

Ciliary epithelium

Basal lamina (Bruch's membrane)

Stratum vasculosum (stroma)

Ciliary muscle

Supraciliary lamina

Fig. 18-5. Part of a meridional section through the **ciliary body.** H and E. x120.

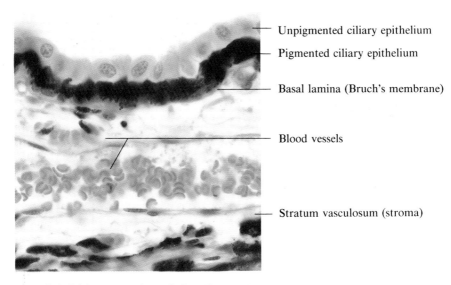

Unpigmented ciliary epithelium

Pigmented ciliary epithelium

Basal lamina (Bruch's membrane)

Blood vessels

Stratum vasculosum (stroma)

Fig. 18-6. High power view of the **ciliary epithelium** and underlying ciliary stroma. H and E. x540.

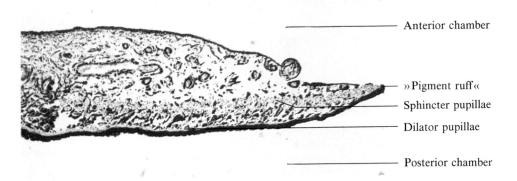

Anterior chamber

»Pigment ruff«
Sphincter pupillae
Dilator pupillae

Posterior chamber

Fig. 18-7. Meridional section through the **iris.** H and E. x75.

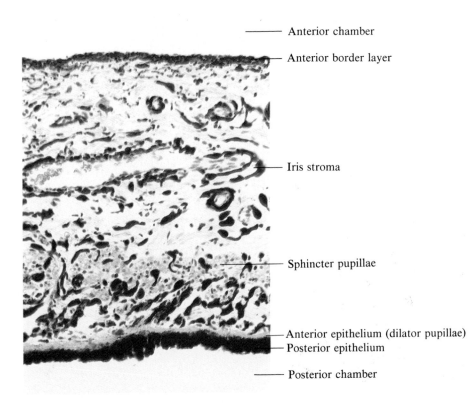

Anterior chamber
Anterior border layer

Iris stroma

Sphincter pupillae

Anterior epithelium (dilator pupillae)
Posterior epithelium

Posterior chamber

Fig. 18-8. Meridional section through the **iris** seen at somewhat higher power. H and E. x210.

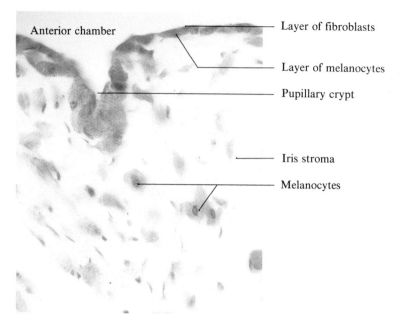

Anterior chamber

Layer of fibroblasts

Layer of melanocytes

Pupillary crypt

Iris stroma

Melanocytes

Fig. 18-9. High power view of the anterior part of the **iris.** Note the exceedingly thin layer of flattened fibroblasts towards the anterior chamber. H and E. x440.

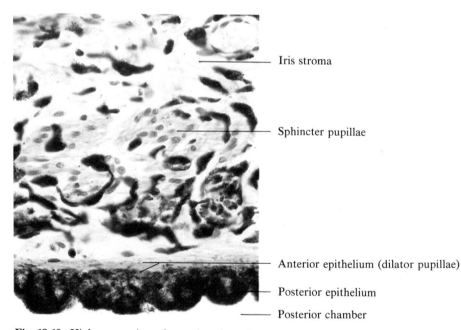

Iris stroma

Sphincter pupillae

Anterior epithelium (dilator pupillae)

Posterior epithelium

Posterior chamber

Fig. 18-10. High power view of a section through the posterior part of the **iris.** H and E. x450.

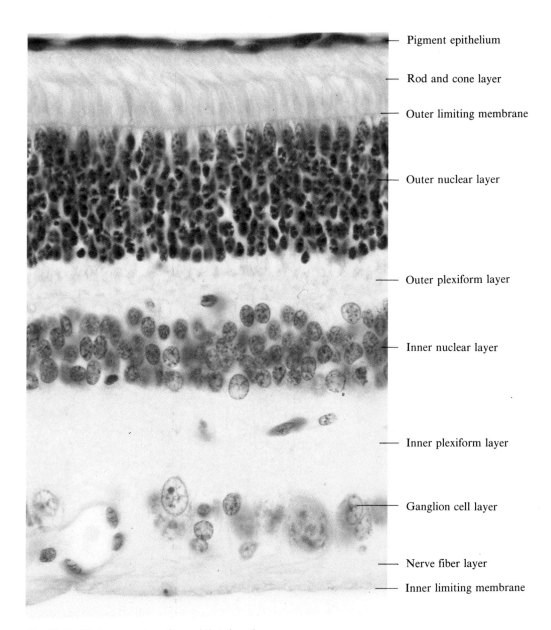

Pigment epithelium

Rod and cone layer

Outer limiting membrane

Outer nuclear layer

Outer plexiform layer

Inner nuclear layer

Inner plexiform layer

Ganglion cell layer

Nerve fiber layer

Inner limiting membrane

Fig. 18-11. High power view of a meridional section through the **retina.** H and E. x810.

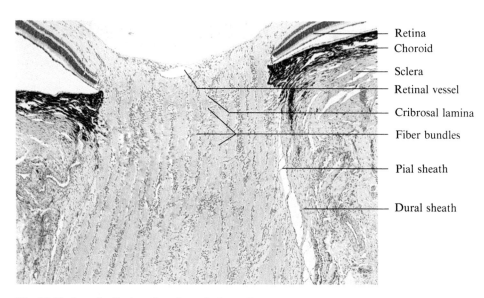

Fig. 18-12. Longitudinal section through the **optic nerve** where it enters the eyeball, that is, corresponding to the **optic disk.** H and E. x45.

Retina
Choroid
Sclera
Retinal vessel
Cribrosal lamina
Fiber bundles
Pial sheath
Dural sheath

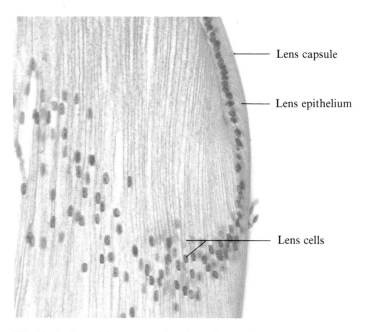

Fig. 18-13. Part of the **equator of the lens.** H and E. x275.

Lens capsule
Lens epithelium
Lens cells

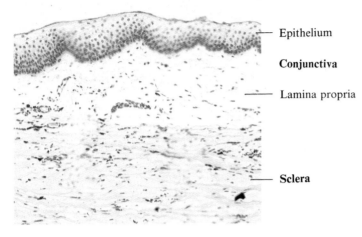

Fig. 18-14. Meridional section through part of the **ocular conjunctiva.** H and E. x110.

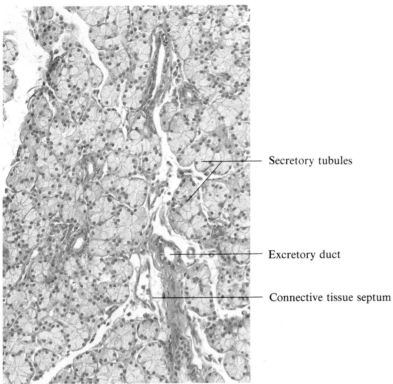

Fig. 18-15. Part of the **lacrimal gland.** H and E. x190.

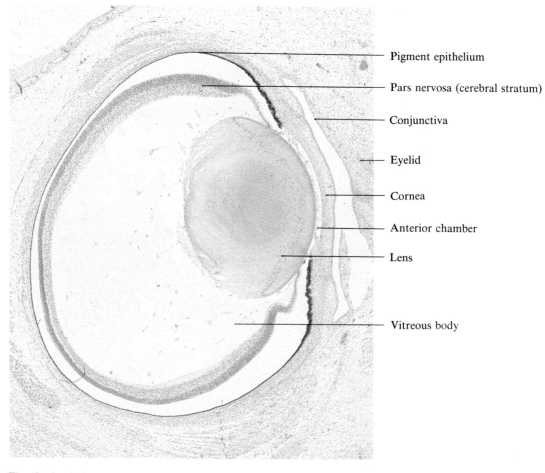

Fig. 18-16. Meridional section through the **primordium of an eye** from a human fetus in the third fetal month. H and E. x32.

CHAPTER 19

The Ear

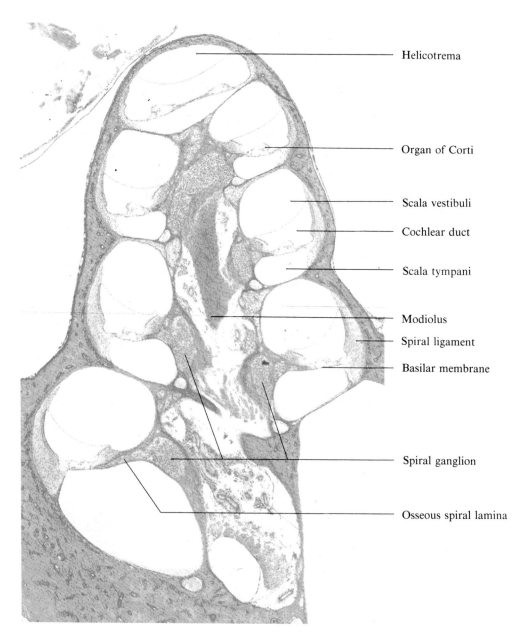

Helicotrema

Organ of Corti

Scala vestibuli

Cochlear duct

Scala tympani

Modiolus

Spiral ligament

Basilar membrane

Spiral ganglion

Osseous spiral lamina

Fig. 19-1. Section through the **cochlea** of a guinea pig. H and E. x37.

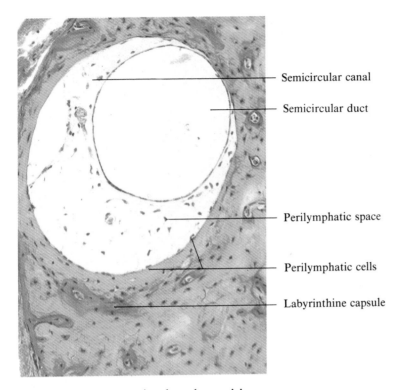

Semicircular canal

Semicircular duct

Perilymphatic space

Perilymphatic cells

Labyrinthine capsule

Fig. 19-2. Transverse section through a **semicircular canal.** H and E. x180.

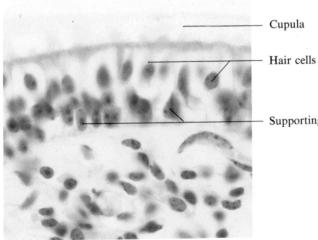

Cupula

Hair cells

Supporting cells

Fig. 19-3. High power view of the specialized receptor epithelium of a **crista ampullaris** of the vestibular labyrinth. H and E. x735.

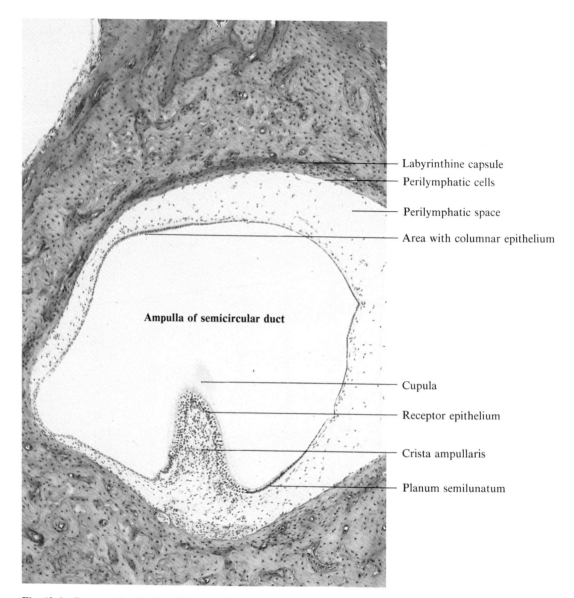

Labyrinthine capsule

Perilymphatic cells

Perilymphatic space

Area with columnar epithelium

Ampulla of semicircular duct

Cupula

Receptor epithelium

Crista ampullaris

Planum semilunatum

Fig. 19-4. Cross sectional view of the **ampulla of a semicircular duct.** H and E. x90.

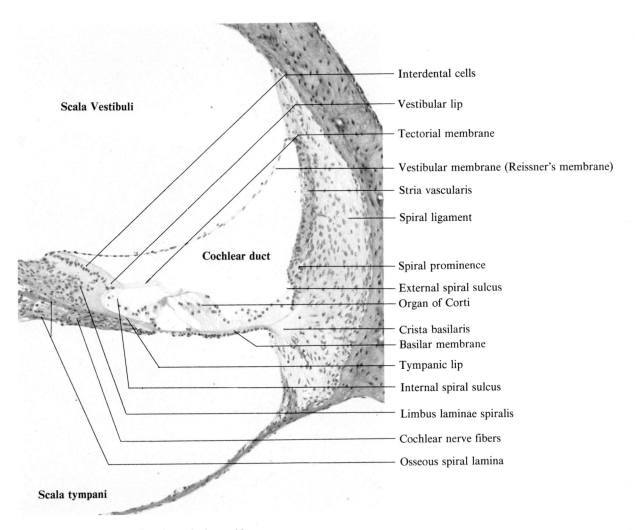

Scala Vestibuli

Cochlear duct

Scala tympani

Interdental cells

Vestibular lip

Tectorial membrane

Vestibular membrane (Reissner's membrane)

Stria vascularis

Spiral ligament

Spiral prominence

External spiral sulcus

Organ of Corti

Crista basilaris

Basilar membrane

Tympanic lip

Internal spiral sulcus

Limbus laminae spiralis

Cochlear nerve fibers

Osseous spiral lamina

Fig. 19-5. Transverse section through the **cochlear duct.** H and E. x130.

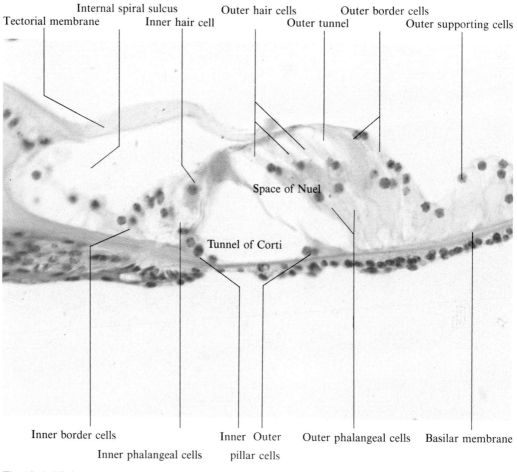

Internal spiral sulcus — Outer hair cells — Outer border cells
Tectorial membrane — Inner hair cell — Outer tunnel — Outer supporting cells

Space of Nuel

Tunnel of Corti

Inner border cells — Inner Outer — Outer phalangeal cells — Basilar membrane
Inner phalangeal cells — pillar cells

Fig. 19-6. High power view of a transverse section through the cochlear duct showing the **organ of Corti**. H and E. x440.

Index

Root canal, of tooth, 107
Root, of tooth, 107
Root sheath, inner, of hair, 93, 94
  outer, of hair, 93, 94

S
Saccus alveolaris, 139
Salivary glands, 100–103
  of lip, 98
Salivary (striated) ducts, 25, 101, 102, 103
Salpinx, 175, 176
Satellite cells, perineuronal, 61
Scala tympani, 216, 219
Scala vestibuli, 216, 219
Schmidt-Lanterman clefts, 59
Schwann cells, 59, 60
Sclera, 206, 207, 213
Scleral stroma, 206
Sebaceous glands, 22, 90, 93, 95, 98
Secondary follicles, of ovaries, 168, 171
Secondary follicle, wall of, 172
Secondary spermatocytes, 184
Secretory epithelial sheath, 23
Secretory granules, 12, 26
Secretory mechanism, apocrine, 22
  holocrine, 22
  merocrine, 22
  Secretory phase, of endometrium, 179
  Semicircular canal, 217
  Semicircular duct, 18, 217, 218
Seminal vesicles, 191
Seminiferous epithelium, 183, 184
Seminiferous tubules, 182, 183, 185, 186
Sensory nerve endings, encapsulated, 62
Sensory neurons, of spinal ganglion, 57
Septum penis, 193
Serous acini, 100, 101, 102
Serous demilunes, 102, 103
Sertoli cells, 184
Sheathed capillary, of spleen, 86
Silver impregnation, of nerve cells, 57
  of reticular fibers, 28, 33, 83, 127
Silver staining, of argentaffin cells, 121
Simple columnar epithelium, 18, 19
Simple cuboidal epithelium, 18
Simple sensory corpuscle, 62
Simple squamous epithelium, 18
Sinuses, of lymph nodes, 80, 81, 82, 83
Sinusoids, of adrenal cortex, 164
  of bone marrow, 38
  of hypophysis, 156
  of liver, 73, 126, 127
  of spleen, 84, 86
Skeletal muscle, 50, 52, 53
  microvasculature of, 53
  of tongue, 99, 100
Skeletal tissues, 42–48
Skin, 90–96
  thick, 90, 91, 92
  thin, 90, 92, 93
Small intestinal mucosa, 19, 22, 23, 116
Small intestine, 115, 116, 117, 118
  endocrine cells of mucosa of, 117

general structure of wall of, 115
  lamina propria of, 12, 31, 117
  mucosa of, 19, 22, 23, 116, 117
Smooth muscle, 10, 50, 51
Smooth muscle cells, 10, 50, 51
  of myometrium, 180
Soma (cell body), of nerve cell, 56
Somatostatin-producing (D) cells, of islets of
  Langerhans, 124
  of small intestinal mucosa, 117
Space of Disse, 127
Space of Nuel, of organ of Corti, 220
Spermatic cord, 190
Spermatids, 184
Spermatogonia, 184
Spermatozoon, 185
Sphincter pupillae muscle, 209, 210
Spinae, dendritic, 56
Spinal ganglion, 60, 61
Spiral artery, of endometrium, 178
Spiral ganglion, 216
Spiral lamina, osseous, 216, 219
Spiral ligament, of cochlear labyrinth, 216, 219
Spiral prominence, of cochlear labyrinth, 219
Spleen, 84–86
  general structure of, 84
Splenic cords (of Billroth), 84, 86
Splenic sinusoids, 84, 86
Spongiocytes, of adrenal cortex, 164
Squamous epithelium, simple, 18
  stratified, keratinized, 20, 91
    nonkeratinized, 19, 20
Stellate reticulum, of primordium of tooth, 104,
  105, 106
Stem cells, 39
Stereocilia, of ductus deferens, 189
  of ductus epididymidis, 19, 188
Stomach, 110–114
  gastric pits of, 112, 113
  gastrin-producing (G) cells of, 114
  general structure of wall of, 111
  mucosa of body of, 10, 112, 113
  mucosa of pyloric part of, 114
  surface epithelium of, 18, 23, 112
Stratified columnar epithelium, 20
Stratified squamous epithelium, keratinized, 20,
  91
  nonkeratinized, 19, 20
  of tonsillary crypt, 87
Stratum basale, of epidermis, 91
Stratum corneum, of epidermis, 91
Stratum disjunctum, of epidermis, 91
Stratum granulosum, of epidermis, 91, 92
Stratum lucidum, of epidermis, 91
Stratum papillare, of dermis, 91
Stratum reticulare, of dermis, 91
Stratum spinosum, of epidermis, 91, 92
Stratum vasculosum (stroma), of ciliary body,
  208
Stria vascularis, of cochlear labyrinth, 219
Stroma, of cornea, 19, 206
Subcapsular sinus, of lymph nodes, 80, 81
Subcutaneous layer, 90